EMERGENCY MEDICINE 1001

EMERGENCY MEDICINE 1001

One Thousand and One Clicks Away

Sergey M. Motov, MD

Attending Emergency Physician
Department of Emergency Medicine
Maimonides Medical Center
Brooklyn, New York

Library of Congress Control Number:	2007905059
ISBN: Softcover	978-1-4257-7982-5

This book was printed in the United States of America.

To order additional copies of this book, contact:
Xlibris Corporation
1-888-795-4274
www.Xlibris.com
Orders@Xlibris.com
40856

CONTENTS

Foreword

Although browsing the Web can be an enjoyable pastime for some, emergency medicine physicians often require accurate and dependable information rapidly. Dr. Motov, a respected emergency medicine attending physician, initially created *Emergency Medicine 1001* for his EM residents and attending colleagues. It was an instant success! With the well-organized index, locating exact information on specific EM topics is but a few clicks away! *Emergency Medicine 1001* provides a comprehensive data bank of Web sites to access your immediate clinical, educational, or research needs. As emergency physicians' time is always of value, whether it is shortening the interval to patient care or optimizing your free time, using *Emergency Medicine 1001* will make a difference!

Carl Ramsay, MD
FACEP

Preface

Dear Colleagues:

I would like to introduce you to the *Emergency Medicine 1001*, the ultimate guide to emergency medicine on the Web. This is an attempt to put together a compilation of online resources dedicated to emergency medicine. The list is extensive and includes 1,001 links. To my knowledge, this is the biggest resource of most current and updated Web sites.

It is impossible to imagine ER doctors going through the shift without even once accessing or looking up something online. The guide is designed to make the navigation through the Web easy and efficient.

I hope that you will find these links useful and applicable to your practice, whether you are an attending, a resident, a nurse, or medical student.

Obviously, it is impossible to include every single Web site dedicated to EM, but this is a first attempt to summarize the best available resources for emergency physicians. In the long run, using your input, we will be able to create even a larger list.

Thank you all in advance for taking your time to go through the guide. I will gladly accept any comments, suggestions, and, especially, additional Web sites that you might provide. The replies should be sent to smotov@yahoo.com.

Enjoy the journey to the world of EM!

Sergey M. Motov, MD

1. Acknowledgment

1. **Maimonides Medical Center (Department of Emergency Medicine).** Sweet home.
   http://www.mmc-em.org/

2. **EMedConcepts (Emerging Medical Concepts).** Leadership outlook in emergency medicine and developing hospital-based leaders in hospital-based medical practices.
   http://www.emedconcepts.com/

3. **EMCrit (Emergency Medicine and ED Critical Care).** Based on evidences and references—the best of the best!
   http://www.emcrit.org/

2. Bookmarks

1. **American Heart Association.** Scientific statements, all the heart stuff.
   http://www.americanheart.org/

2. **Attract.** Ask any questions you want.
   http://www.attract.wales.nhs.uk/

3. **Bandolier (Evidence Based Thinking About Health Care).**
   http://www.jr2.ox.ac.uk/bandolier/index.html

4. **Bayesian Analysis.** Remember the statistics.
   http://www.intmed.mcw.edu/clincalc/bayes.html

5. **Center for Evidence-Based Medicine.** Speaks for itself.
   http://www.cebm.utoronto.ca/

6. **Clinical Trial Results.** Great resource of information.
   http://www.clinicaltrialresults.org/

7. **EBM & Clinical Research Workstation**. Great tools in understanding research.
   http://www.msugrem.org/ebm/

8. **Evidence Based Medical Tool Kit.** You've got to use them.
   http://www.med.ualberta.ca/ebm/ebm.htm

9. **How to Read a Medical Journal Article.** Great site.
   http://www.childrens-mercy.org/stats/journal.asp

10. **InfoPOEMs.** Provides clinicians with the best available evidence as they practice.
    http://www.infopoems.com/

11. **Research-Based Web Design and Usability Guidelines.** Take a look.
    http://www.usability.gov/pdfs/guidelines.html

12. **The Cochrane Library**. Source to use!
    http://www.update-software.com/publications/cochrane/

13. **CogPsychTutor (Cognitive Psychology Tutor)**. Great help for clinicians.
    http://teach.psy.uga.edu/CogPsychTutor/

14. **National Guideline Clearinghouse.** I love this site!
    http://www.guideline.gov/

15. **No Free Lunch**. What about those Representatives.
    http://www.nofreelunch.org/

16. **PREtest Consult.** Are you sure?
    http://www.pretestconsult.com/

17. **Web M & M (Morbidity and Mortality Rounds on the Web).** You have to read this!
    http://www.webmm.ahrq.gov/

18. **Aggravated DocSurg.** Incoherent ramblings and flatulence from a general surgeon.
    http://www.docsurg.blogspot.com/

19. **GruntDoc.** For those who grunts.
    http://www.gruntdoc.com/

20. **Medscape.** Great information on the site.
    http://www.medscape.com/

21. **UpToDate.** One of my favorite—needs subscription.
    http://www.uptodate.com/

22. **PubMed.** Great search engine!
    http://www.ncbi.nlm.nih.gov/sites/entrez

23. **Medical Education Online (MEO).** A forum for disseminating information on educating physicians.
    http://www.med-ed-online.org/

24. **AHC Media LLC (American Health Consultant Online).** Part of the site includes nice EM information.
    http://www.ahcpub.com/

25. **MedConnect (An Online Resource for Health Professionals).**
    http://www.medconnect.com/

26. **ScHARR Information Resources Bookmarks.** Great resource for pretty much everything—got to look!
    http://www.shef.ac.uk/scharr/ir/abookmrk.html

27. **Doctor's Guide (Global Edition).** Doctor's guide to the Internet—it is a guide must-have!
    http://www.docguide.com/

28. **Emergency.com (Emergency Response and Research Institute).** Includes crisis, conflict, and emergency service news, analysis, and reference.
    http://www.emergency.com/

29. **Land of Medical Links: by Joe Buenker.** A very useful site with lots of information.
    http://www.west.asu.edu/jbuenke/medicine/

30. **McGraw-Hill's Access Medicine (Harrison Online).** The best minds in medicine—requires subscription.
    http://www.accessmedicine.com/

31. **MedInfoRus (Medical Information in Russian).** For those who are interested in Russian medical information.
    http://medinforus.homestead.com/MedInfoRus.html

32. **DB's Medical Rants.** An academic general internist comments on medical issues and the current state of medicine.
http://www.medrants.com/

33. **Emergency Medical Doctor**. Excellent site for EM physicians—a must-read!
http://emergmeddoc.com/

34. **Medical News Feeds.** Medical news and Weblog aggregator—a must-read site!
http://www.medlogs.com/

35. **Medpundit.** A commentary on medical news by a practicing physician.
http://medpundit.blogspot.com/

36. **MedCases.** Effective, efficient, and engaging medical education.
http://www.medcases.com/

37. **Journal Club Storage Bank.** An electronic repository.
http://www.ebem.org/jcb/journalclubbank.html

38. **MDchoice.com.** The ultimate medical search engine.
http://www.mdchoice.com/index.asp

3. Airway Management

1. **The Airway Institute.** A place where to start.
    http://airwayinstitute.com/

2. **Dr. Magboul Airway Page.** My favorite site—a must-read site! A subscription to MSSN is required.
    http://groups.msn.com/DrMAGBOULAIRWAYPAGE/

3. **Evaluation of the Emergency Airway.** A must-read!
    http://web.archive.org/web/20000615202131/anesthesiology.
    mc.vanderbilt.edu/resweb/eamg/Eamg2.htm

4. **Indirect Tracheal Intubation.** A very meticulous review.
    http://web.archive.org/web/20000311074614/anesthesiology.
    mc.vanderbilt.edu/resweb/eamg/EAMG4.htm

5. **The Use of Pharmacologic Agents in Airway Management.**
    http://web.archive.org/web/20000615113220/anesthesiology.
    mc.vanderbilt.edu/resweb/eamg/EAMG7.htm

6. **Fiberoptic Intubation and the Difficult Airway.**
    http://web.archive.org/web/20000229040535/anesthesiology.
    mc.vanderbilt.edu/resweb/eamg/EAMG6.HTM

7. **Pediatric Airway Management.**
    http://web.archive.org/web/20000615174318/anesthesiology.
    mc.vanderbilt.edu/resweb/eamg/EAMG9.htm

8. **Management of the Difficult Airway.** Great slide show. Keep it handy, but you have to have access from Yale University.
http://gasnet.med.yale.edu/airway/title.htm

9. **The Pediatric Video.** Optical intubation stylet.
http://www.ispub.com/ostia/index.php?xmlFilePath=journals/ija/vol2n4/vois.xml

10. **The Pediatric Airway.** A slide show on the practical approach to airway management.
http://www.gavinmorrison.com/presentations/airway/airway.htm

11. **Canadian Journal of Anesthesia (Airway resources on the Internet: Part 2).** Lots of useful links.
http://www.cja-jca.org/cgi/content/full/47/4/375

12. **The Airway Site.** The airway management definitive site!
http://www.theairwaysite.com/

13. **Difficult Airway Society Guidelines.**
http://www.guideline.gov/summary/summary.aspx?view_id=1&doc_id=6183

14. **Internet Journal of Airway Management.** Articles related to airway management in anesthesia, intensive care, and emergency medicine.
http://www.adair.at/ijam/default.asp

15. **Use of Percutaneous Transtracheal Jet Ventilation(PTJV) during Difficult airway Management.** Here is the difficult intubation.
http://www.ispub.com/ostia/index.php?xmlFilePath=journals/ijeicm/vol3n1/ptjv.xml

16. **The Combitube.** Absolutely a must-read site!
http://www.meduniwien.ac.at/combitube/combit1.html

17. **Street Level Airway Management Society.** Insanely great site!
http://www.airwayeducation.com/

18. **Fiberoptic Intubation.** Everything you need to know.
    http://faculty.washington.edu/pcolley/

19. **Virtual Anesthesia Textbook (The Airway Management).** A must-read site!
    http://www.virtual-anaesthesia-textbook.com/vat/intubation.html

20. **Endotracheal Intubation by Direct Laryngoscopy.** Here we start!
    http://www.thoracic.org/sections/clinical-information/critical-care/atlas-of-critical-care-procedures/procedures/endotracheal-intubation-by-direct-laryngoscopy.cfm

21. **Airway Management.** In slides.
    http://anes.usuhs.mil/Medical/AIRWAY_files/

22. **Difficult Intubation.** A very good slide collection.
    http://www.palmer.net.au/talks/cab_diffintub/default.htm

23. **Difficult Airway Management (Action Plan for Airway Problems from Hell!).** Really are!
    http://www.enw.org/AirwayHell.htm

24. **Prediction and Management of Difficult Tracheal Intubation.**
    http://www.nda.ox.ac.uk/wfsa/html/u09/u09_025.htm

25. **The Airway Carnival (Laryngeal Mask Airway).**
    http://www.airwaycarnival.com/LMA.htm

26. **Emergency Nursing World! (Fix This Airway!)**
    http://enw.org/FixThisAirway.htm

27. **Upper Airway Management—Application of New Technologies.**
    http://www.anesthesia.org/winterlude/wl97/w_airway.html

28. **Austrian Difficult Airway/Intubation Registry.**
    http://www.adair.at/start.asp?Lan=E

29. **The Dilemma of Airway Assessment and Evaluation.** By Dr. Magboul.
    http://www.ispub.com/ostia/index.php?xmlFilePath=journals/ija/
    vol10n1/airway.xml

30. **Tracheostomy Care.** Everything that you need in your practice.
    http://www.northeastcenter.com/links_ventilator_tracheostomy.
    htm

4. Clinical Tools

1. **Antibiotic-Consult.com.** Good-bye Stanford!
   http://www.antibiotic-consult.com/

2. **U.S. Food and Drug Administration (Drug Shortages Resources).**
   Please read.
   http://www.fda.gov/cder/drug/shortages/

3. **2007 EMRA Antibiotics Guide.** Keep it in your pocket.
   http://www2.acep.org/bookstore/index.cfm?go=product.detail&
   id=396

4. **Gray's Anatomy.** Good to remember.
   http://www.bartleby.com/107/

5. **Johns Hopkins Division of Infectious Diseases Antibiotic Guide
   (ABX Guide).** Good clinical source.
   http://www.hopkins-abxguide.org/

6. **MD Consult Books Search.** You will like it.
   http://www.mdconsult.com/

7. **MEDLINE Search.** The best as ever has been.
   http://www.nlm.nih.gov/databases/databases_medline.html

8. **The Medical Algorithms Project.** Any computation, formula, survey,
   or lookup table that is useful in health care.
   http://www.medal.org/

9. **MedCalc.** The medical calculator with most complete resource.
    http://www.med-ia.ch/medcalc/

10. **MerckMedicus.** Key to the medical Internet.
    http://www.merckmedicus.com/

11. **OnsiteHealth (The Mount Sinai Medical Center).** Welcome to the partner's site.
    http://www.msonsitehealth.org/

12. **National Center for Emergency Medicine Informatics (Emergency Medicine on the Web).** Have to have it!
    http://www.ncemi.org/

13. **Pneumonia Severity Index Calculator.** A useful tool.
    http://pda.ahrq.gov/clinic/psi/psi.htm

14. **Nursebob's MICU/CCU Survival Guide (Critical Care Concepts) APACHE II.** Useful to calculate.
    http://rnbob.tripod.com/apachescore.htm

15. **Acid-Base Tutorial.** Absolutely the best site.
    http://www.acid-base.com/

16. **USC Physiology ACID-BASE Center.** Everything you need to know.
    http://ppn.med.sc.edu/watson/Acidbase/Acidbase.htm

17. **Web Pages that Perform Statistical Calculations!**
    http://statpages.org/

18. **Online Clinical Calculators.** Medical site
    http://www.intmed.mcw.edu/clincalc.html

19. **The Statistics Homepage.** For those who is in Statistics.
    http://www.statsoft.com/textbook/stathome.html

20. **PubMed Tutorial.** For novice people on the Internet.
    http://www.chu-rouen.fr/documed/pmeeng.html

21. **Diagnostic Test Calculator.**
    http://araw.mede.uic.edu/cgi-bin/testcalc.pl

22. **ACLS Megacode Simulator.**
    http://www.mdchoice.com/cyberpt/acls/acls.asp

23. **Pediatric Advanced Cardiac Life Support Megacode Simulator.**
    http://www.mdchoice.com/cyberpt/pals/pals.asp

24. **ClinicalExam.com.** Everything you need to know!
    http://www.clinicalexam.com/

25. **Perinatology.com—Drugs in Pregnancy and Breastfeeding.**
    http://www.perinatology.com/exposures/druglist.htm

26. **NetPharmacology—Cardiovascular Pharmacology Lecture notes.**
    Amazing lectures!
    http://lysine.pharm.utah.edu/netpharm/netpharm_00/notes.html

27. **Cardiology in Critical Care (Transvenous Pacemaker Insertion).**
    Great resource!
    http://rnbob.tripod.com/transven.htm

5. Decision/Prediction Rules

1. National Emergency Medicine Informatics (NCEMI).
   http://www.ncemi.org/

2. Clinical Predictors Rules.
   http://www.mssm.edu/medicine/general-medicine/ebm/#cpr

3. TIMI Risk Calculator for Unstable Angina.
   http://www.timi.org/files/riskscore/ua_calculator.htm

4. TIMI Risk Calculator for Acute MI.
   http://www.timi.org/files/riskscore/mi_calculator.htm

5. The Heart Failure Mortality Prediction Rules.
   http://www.ccort.ca/CHFriskmodel.aspx

6. Ottawa Health Research Institute—Clinical Decision Rules.
   http://www.ohri.ca/programs/clinical_epidemiology/OHDEC/
   clinical.asp

7. Lab Tests Online.
   http://www.labtestsonline.org/index.html

6. Critical Care

1. **American Thoracic Society—Critical Care.**
   http://www.thoracic.org/sections/clinical-information/critical-care/index.html

2. **James Allen, M.D. Home Page.** Critical care guys page that contains information for medical students and residents.
   http://home.columbus.rr.com/allen/

3. **Evidence Based Decisions Making.** Critical care—great approach to EBM.
   http://www.evidencebased.net/

4. **Pulmonary Artery Catheter Education Project (PACEP).** Here comes your PCWP.
   http://www.pacep.org/

5. **Critical Care Medicine Tutorials.** The best site ever!
   http://www.ccmtutorials.com

6. **American College of Emergency Physicians.** Check critical care section.
   http://www.acep.org/

7. **Critical Care.** See forum with international resources.
   http://www.ccforum.com/home

8. **Society of Critical Care Medicine.**
   http://www.sccm.org/

9. **European Society of Intensive Care Medicine.**
   http://www.esicm.org/

10. **International Sepsis Forum.** Initiative to focus solely on management
    of patients with severe sepsis.
    http://www.sepsisforum.org/

11. **MedBioWorld**. That is all you need to have!
    http://www.medbioworld.com/

12. **Anaesthetist.com.** The world of anesthesia for critical care—great site
    for CCM.
    http://www.anaesthetist.com/

13. **Trauma.org.** See for yourself!
    http://www.trauma.org/

14. **Sepsis.com.** Pretty much everything you should know.
    http://www.sepsis.com/

15. **Critical Care Nutrition.** Useful site for ICU rotation.
    http://www.criticalcarenutrition.com

16. **Capnography.com.** Everything you need to know.
    http://www.capnography.com/

17. **VentWorld.com. Everything you need to know about mechanical
    ventilation.**
    http://www.ventworld.com/

18. **The Internet Journal of Emergency and Intensive Care Medicine.**
    http://www.uam.es/departamentos/medicina/anesnet/journals/
    ijeicm.htm

19. **Early Goal Directed Therapy: A Collaborative Protocol.** Great audio
    lecture!
    http://www.edwards.com/products/mininvasive/levypvideo.htm

20. **The MUST Guide to Sepsis.** A must-have site!
    http://sepsis.bidmc.harvard.edu/Content/start_frameset.htm

21. **Intensive Care On-line Network.** Great database.
    http://www.intensivecareonline.com/

22. **Critical Care.** It's Showtime!
    http://critical-care.sourceforge.net/

23. **National Registry of Cardiopulmonary Resuscitation.**
    http://www.nrcpr.org/

24. **Drug Dosages in Medical Emergencies.**
    http://www.priory.co.uk/emerg.htm

25. **Critical Care and Shock.** You must read it!
    http://www.criticalcareshock.org/index.asp

26. **Intensive Care, Critical Care, and Emergency Medicine Journals.**
    http://www.medbioworld.com/

27. **Early Goal Directed Therapy: A Collaborative Protocol.** A PowerPoint
    presentation by Dr. Levy.
    http://www.edwards.com/products/mininvasive/levypvideo.htm

7. Continuous Medical Education (CME)

1. **CME download.com.**
   http://www.cmedownload.com/

2. **Oakstone Medical Publishing.** Practical reviews for MDs. A gateway
   to continuing education credit.
   http://www.oakstonemedical.com/

3. **CMEonly.com**. This might take long time to load.
   http://www.cmeonly.com/

4. **CME List (Online Continuing Medical Education).** Useful site.
   http://www.cmelist.com/

5. **Alliance for Continuing Medical Education-ACME.** International
   association of CME professionals.
   http://www.acme-assn.org/

6. **Society for Academic Continuing Medical Education-SACME.** For
   academic continuing education.
   http://www.sacme.org/index.html/

7. **Emergency Medicine Continuous Certification.** Part of ABEM site.
   http://www.abem.org/public/portal/alias__Rainbow/lang__en-US/
   tabID__3421/DesktopDefault.aspx

8. **Center for Emergency Medical Education.**
   http://www.ceme.org/

9. **Emergency Medicine Education Systems.** Great board review and ELISA review!
    http://www.emedsinc.com/

10. **Essentials of Emergency Medicine.** The Center for Medical Education, Inc.
    http://ccme.org/

11. **Institute for Emergency Medical Education.** Nonprofit foundation dedicated to excellence in medical education.
    http://www.ieme.com/

12. **The Center for Emergency Medical Education (CEME).** Educational opportunities for emergency physicians
    http://www.ceme.org

8. Evidence Based Medicine

1. **The Bandolier.** EB thinking of health care.
   http://www.jr2.ox.ac.uk/bandolier

2. **Evidence-Based Medicine**. Research in the field of health information science.
   http://hiru.mcmaster.ca/

3. **Evidence-Based on-call.**
   http://www.eboncall.co.uk/

4. **The Evidence-Based Emergency medicine**. Great site.
   http://www.ebem.org/index.php

5. **The User Guide to EBM.**
   http://www.cche.net/usersguides/main.asp

6. **The EBM On-call.** Enjoy your journey.
   http://www.eboncall.org/

7. **Dr. Chris Cates EBM**. Fun to navigate.
   http://www.nntonline.net/

8. **The BMJ Update.**
   http://bmjupdates.mcmaster.ca/index.asp

9. **User's Guide to Medical Literature.**
   http://www.usersguides.org/

10. **Emergency Medicine Based on Evidences**. Absolutely the best!
http://www.emcrit.org/

11. **Center for Evidence Based Medicine.**
http://www.cebm.utoronto.ca/

12. **EBM Toolkit.** Identifying, assessing, and applying relevant evidence for better health care decision making.
http://www.med.ualberta.ca/ebm/ebm.htm

13. **Evidence-Based Medicine**. Nice general overview
http://www.herts.ac.uk/lis/subjects/health/ebm.htm

14. **Health Services/Technology Assessment Text (HSTAT).** Provide health information and support health care decision making.
http://www.ncbi.nlm.nih.gov/books/bv.fcgi?rid=hstat

15. **Center for Evidence-based Medicine.** Founded by Oxford.
http://www.cebm.net

16. **Netting the Evidence (A ScHARR Introduction to Evidence Based Practice on the Internet).** Useful tool for approaching medical literature.
http://www.shef.ac.uk/scharr/ir/netting

17. **CRITICAL APPRAISAL. User Guides to the Medical Literature (JAMA).** List of sites for EBM—my favorite.
http://www.shef.ac.uk/scharr/ir/userg.html

18. **ClinicalTrials.gov.** Provides regularly updated information about clinical research in human volunteers—great site.
http://www.clinicaltrials.gov

19. **EBM & Clinical Research Workstation.**
http://msugrem.org/ebm

20. **CATwalk.** Guided walk through the process of doing critically appraised topic.
http://www.library.ualberta.ca/subject/healthsciences/catwalk/index.cfm

21. **BestBETs Web site**. Rapid evidence-based answers to real-life clinical questions.
    http://www.bestbets.org

22. **Introduction to Evidence Based Medicine at McGill.**
    http://www.health.library.mcgill.ca/ebm

23. **Centre for Health Evidence.**
    http://www.cche.net/

24. **Evidence-based Medicine Resource Center.**
    http://www.ebmny.org/

25. **Users' Guides Interactive.** An online tool to guide clinicians in the appraisal and application of evidence into their everyday practice.
    http://www.usersguides.org/

26. **Turning Research into Practice.** The Internet's leading resources for evidence-based medicine.
    http://www.tripdatabase.com/index.html

27. **Clinical Guidelines for Care of the Emergency Patient.**
    http://www.ed.bmc.org/emguidelines/guideem.html

9. Electrocardiography (EKG)

1. **ECG Library.** A very useful site.
    http://www.ecglibrary.com/

2. **Albany Medical Review.** EKG and x-ray cases.
    http://www.amc.edu/amr/archives

3. **Cardiology Cases.** Great site.
    http://www.clinicalcases.blogspot.com

4. **EKG Learning Center.** Absolutely the best must-read site!
    http://medlib.med.utah.edu/kw/ecg/

5. **EKG Cases Files.** Great educational site.
    http://www.angelfire.com/nj4/ekg/casemenu.html

6. **Heart Rhythm Society.** Speaks for itself!
    http://www.hrsonline.org/

7. **Martindale's Virtual Cardiology.** Awesome site.
    http://www.martindalecenter.com

8. **Emergency EKG Online Tutorial.** Must-have site!
    http://www.emedu.org/ecg

9. **Essentials EKG for Physicians.** Amazing site!
    http://themdsite.com/?gclid=CLWO87L6xIoCFQFRUAodZzyfew

10. **EKG strip Evaluation.** Oriented for nurses but surely deserves your attention.
    http://www.rnceus.com/

11. **eMedicine ECG Cases.**
    http://www.emedicine.com/ekgotwindexbytitle.html

12. **ECG on-line Teaching Module.**
    http://www.emedu.org/ecg/

13. **The Twelve-Lead Electrocardiography of Myocardial Infarction.**
    http://sprojects.mmi.mcgill.ca/heart/mimenu.html

14. **Basics of EKG Interpretation.** A programmed study.
    http://nps.freeservers.com/ekg.htm

15. **EKG Chapter.**
    http://www.fpnotebook.com/CVCh3.htm

16. **ECG Rounds (MDchoice.com). Great selections of EKGs.**
    http://www.mdchoice.com/ekg/ekg.asp

17. **EKG for the beginners.** Top sites selection.
    http://www.searchdoppler.com/ekg.htm

18. **EKG Images database. EKG heaven!**
    http://images.ask.com/pictures?o=0&pstart=&qsrc=6&l=dir&q=E kg+Tutorial

10. Emergency Medicine

1.   **ACLS Provider Course.** Straight from AHA.
     http://www.americanheart.org/presenter.jhtml?identifier=3011972

2.   **ACLS on-line.** Great site.
     http://www.ACLS.net/

3.   **American Safety and Health Institute.**
     http://www.ashinstitute.com/

4.   **Updated ACLS Guidelines.** Got to read!
     http://www.medscape.com/viewarticle/536075?rss

5.   **Acute Care, Inc.** Pictures, EKG, and x-rays
     http://www.acutecare.com/

6.   **AMA Doctors Finder.**
     http://webapps.ama-assn.org/doctorfinder/home.html?aps/amahg.
     htm

7.   **American Academy of Pediatrics.**
     http://www.aap.org/

8.   **AAP-Pediatric Emergency Course.**
     http://www.aplsonline.com/

9.   **Advanced Hazmat Life Support.**
     http://www.ahls.org/

10. **American College of Medical Toxicology.**
http://www.acmt.net/main

11. **Agency of Toxic Substances.** Serves the public by using the best science, taking responsive public health actions.
http://www.atsdr.cdc.gov/

12. **Advanced Life Support.** Pediatrics and adults.
http://www.aclsonline.us

13. **Alan Clark's Mind sharpener.** One of the best sites!
http://www.erworld.com/mindsharp

14. **Clark's Emergency Medicine World**. A must-see site.
http://www.erworld.com/

15. **Carol Rivers Board Review.** A must-have site!
http://www.emeeinc.com/

16. **The Emergency Medicine and Primary Care Home Page**. Nice resources!
http://www.pslgroup.com/dg/3a36.htm

17. **Emergency Medicine Harvard—Find The Pathology.** Great site!
http://www.brighamrad.harvard.edu

18. **ER.** Official site for the greatest show!
http://www.nbc.com/ER/

19. **EMedHome.com: my favorite.** Costs few pennies.
http://www.EMedHome.com/

20. **EMED Listserve Archives.** Messaging service.
http://www.ucsf.edu/its/listserv/emed-l/

21. **Emergency Medicine Cyber School.** Good cases.
http://www.mssm.edu/emergmed/cschool.htm

22. **Brown Emergency Medicine Case Reviews.**
www.brown.edu/Administration/Emergency_Medicine/emr/pages/
cases.html

23. **EM Guidemaps (Jeff Mann's).** One of the top sites in my opinion!
http://www.jeffmann.net/

24. **Emergency Medicine on the Web.** Great!
http://www.ncemi.org/

25. **Emergency Department Favorite Sites.** Oh boy, nothing compares to it!
http://www.erstat.com/

26. **EMEDICINE.** I love it!
http://www.emedicine.com/

27. **Emergency Medical Abstracts.** A must-have site!
http://ccme.org/

28. **Emergency Medicine Practice.** I live in this site!
http://www.ebmedpractice.net/

29. **Emergency Medicine Reports**. Great site.
http://www.emronline.com/

30. **Emergency Medicine MDLinx.** Great database.
www.mdlinx.com/emergencymdlinx/index.cfm

31. **EMRap.** Keep rapping!
http://prod2.ccme.org/emrap/

32. **EM Tests.** Part of the CORD site.
http://www.emtests.com/

33. **ER Doc Dot.** Good general overview.
http://www.erdoc.com/

34. **Emergency Medicine Doc.** News, facts, media, and blogging!
http://www.emergmeddoc.com/

35. **Emergency Medicine**. Discussing the specialty.
http://www.erbook.net/

36. **Emergency Medicine Watch.** Well, keep watching!
http://emergency-medicine.jwatch.org/

37. **Medical Matrix.** Clinical medicine resources.
http://www.medmatrix.org/

38. **Emergency Medicine Procedures Online.** A compilation of questions
for preparation for the written and oral board examinations.
http://www.super-memory.com/sml/2003/536.htm

39. **Emergency Medicine Education Online**. Just look at it! Simply the best!
http://www.emedu.org/

40. **The Airway Site**. Got to have it!
http://www.theairwaysite.com/

41. **The Gist of Emergency Medicine.** A must-read site!
http://www.erbook.com/

42. **Weekly Web Review in Emergency Medicine**. Nicely-put-together site.
http://www.wwrem.com/

43. **Common Simple Emergencies**. Quick reference site.
http://www.ncemi.org/cse/contents.htm

44. **Emergency Medicine Alert**. Paid subscription required, monthly issues.
http://www.ramex.com/title.asp?id=9464

45. **ED Legal Letter**. From the perspective of risk management and malpractice
prevention (paid subscription).
http://www.ramex.com/title.asp?id=9460

46. **The National Emergency Board Review.**
http://www.emboards.com/

47. **Finding-the-Path: A Problem-based Guide to Diagnostic Imaging Strategies in the Emergency Room.**
http://brighamrad.harvard.edu/education/online/ftp/FTP.html

48. **The Precise Neurological Examination.** Great tutorial site.
http://endeavor.med.nyu.edu/neurosurgery/index.html

49. **At Emergency.com**. Search engine for ER stuff.
http://atemergency.com/er/

50. **EDSubscriber@ncemi**. A tool for autosubscribing to medical e-mail lists.
http://www.ncemi.org/emergency_medicine/edsubscriber.htm

51. **Web Site Lists**. Large database of medical information.
http://www.angelfire.com/space2/makrada/medical.htm

52. **Emergency Medicine Doc.** Excellent site for EM Physicians—a must-read!
http://emergmeddoc.com/blog

53. **Mr. Hassle's Long Underpants and Other Stories.** A rookie attending physician takes flight in the Rockies.
http://www.docshazam.com

54. **Richard [WINTERS] MD**. An irregularly irregular Weblog by emergency physician geek.
http://www.richardwinters.com/richardwintersmd/

55. **The Gist of Emergency Medicine**. A must-read and must-have site! The management of real or simulated patient encounters.
http://erbook.com/

56. **Acute Care, Inc**. Favorite links for pictures, radiographs, and EKGs. Truly amazing resource.
http://www.acutecare.com/imagelist.htm

57. **Emergency Medicine Cyber School.**
http://www.mssm.edu/emergmed/cschool.htm

58. **The Emergency Medicine Learning & Resource Center (EMLRC).**
http://www.femf.org/

59. **1,200 Emergency Medicine and Urgent Care Jobs in All States.**
http://www.edphysician.com/

60. **Emergency Medicine Case Bank-Mount Sinai.**
http://www.mssm.edu/emergmed/cases/emframe.html

61. **Emergency Medicine Contraception.**
http://ec.princeton.edu/

62. **Emergency Medicine Links at McGill.**
http://www.mcgill.ca/emergency/links/

63. **Emergency Medicine**. Multiple studies involving patient's safety.
http://www.psnet.ahrq.gov/content.aspx?taxonomyID=312

64. **Emergency Medicine Foundation**. Funds emergency medicine research
and education.
http://my.acep.org/site/PageServer?pagename=wp2_about

65. **Emergency Medicine Notebook**. A resource for family practitioners
and everyone else.
http://www.fpnotebook.com/ER.htm

66. **EMR Consultant**. Matches your specific practice profile against database
of EMR manufacturers.
http://www.emrconsultant.com/?source=google&gclid=CObl_d_
4gYoCFRn1gAodJVksNw

67. **Peer View Media Bar—EM Channel.** Doctors guide to EM.
http://www.docguide.com/news/content.nsf/channel?OpenForm&
dt=g&id=48dde4a73e09a969852568880078c249&c= Emergency+
Medicine

68. **The Emergency Medicine Interest Group.** Providing help form those
who interested in EM.
http://southmed.usouthal.edu/emig/resources.html

69. **Emergency Medicine Job Search**. Large data bank.
http://careers.emedmag.com/

70. **Emergency Response and Research Institute.**
    http://www.emergency.com/

71. **Emergency Nursing World.**
    http://enw.org/

72. **Emergency @ Emergency**. Search engine for common emergencies.
    http://atemergency.com/er/

73. **Emergency Medicine Forum**. Students, residents, and attendings.
    http://forums.studentdoctor.net/forumdisplay.php?f=43

74. **Emergency Medicine Physician Assistants**. Quality, affordable emergency
    department coverage.
    http://www.empa.org/

75. **ED Quality Solutions**. Lots of useful links.
    http://www.ed-qual.com/ Emergency_Medicine_Links/clinical_
    links.htm

76. **Emergency Medicine Doctor's Blog.**
    http://www.emergmeddoc.com/

77. **Emergency Medicine Expert Witnesses.** Largest distribution of any
    national expert witness directory.
    http://www.seakexperts.com/static/specialties_index.aspx/
    Emergency_Medicine.html

78. **Emergency Medicine Jobs and Emergency Medicine News.**
    http://www.edsource.com/

79. **Clinical Guidelines for Care of the Emergency Patient.**
    http://www.ed.bmc.org/EMGuidelines/guideEM.html

80. **Emergency Medicine Network (EMNet)**. Multicenter airway research
    collaboration network.
    http://www.emnet-usa.org/emnet_details.htm

81. **Emergency Medicine Researchers International.**
http://www.dwwalsh.com/

82. **Emergency Medicine Cyber School**. Mount Sinai special.
http://www.mssm.edu/emergmed/cschool.htm

83. **Emergency Medicine Consultants**. Provides consulting and staffing solutions for hospitals, urgent care centers, and emergency rooms.
http://www.traumadoctor.org/

84. **Emergency Medicine Education System**. Review courses. (Actually, I have taken this course myself!)
http://www.emedsinc.com/default.cfm

85. **Rosen's Emergency Medicine On-Line**. The best resource ever!
http://www.rosensemergencymedicine.com/authors.cfm

86. **Access Emergency Medicine**. An innovative online service.
http://www.accessem.com/

87. **Studmed.com= for students by students**. Links to EM.
http://www.internet.is/jonasge/sm_clinic_emergencymedicine.htm

88. **Emergency Medicine Forum**. Forum and message board for emergency medicine.
http://www.topix.net/forum/med/emergency-medicine

89. **www.OPEN-ER.com.** An open-source question bank for attending physicians and residents.
http://www.open-er.com/

90. **Emergency Medicine. Global Med Net medical forum.**
http://www.globalmednet.com/forum/emergenc.htm

91. **Emergency Medicine.** Resource for a student from BMJ.
http://www.studentbmj.com/topics/clinical/emergency_medicine.php

92. **Emergency Medicine EMPOD**. Welcome to Medrounds online.
    http://www.medrounds.org/emergency-medicine/

93. **The EMIG Resources.** Emergency Medicine Interest Group online.
    http://southmed.usouthal.edu/emig/resources.html

94. **Emergency Medicine Doctors and Physicians.** Search engine to find
    a doc.
    http://www.healthgrades.com/

95. **Emergency Medicine links-McGill.**
    http://www.mcgill.ca/emergency/links/

96. **Emergency Medicine Medical Illustration, Medical Animation,
    Anatomical Model.**
    http://findlaw.doereport.com/categories.php?CatID=031&A=
    &I=4

97. **Emergency Medicine Internet Resource Page**. Links to many EM sites.
    http://www.cpr.net/specialties/emergency_medicine/

98. **Acute Medicine Simulation Tests Online.**
    http://www.som.soton.ac.uk/emed/

99. **Emergency Medicine Textbooks Online.** An amazing source of
    information.
    http://www.geocities.com/nyerrn/er/books.htm

100. **The Doctor's Page to Medical Humor.** It's Showtime!
     http://www.doctorspage.net/newdr2.asp?cat=Humor

11. Emergency Medicine Potpourri

1. **Adren@line.**
   http://www.adrenaline112.org/

2. **http://www.ampa.org/Airway Cam Technologies.**
   http://www.airwaycam.com/

3. **Anaphylaxis Committee of the AAAAI.**
   http://www.aaaai.org/

4. **Arizona Emergency Med Research Center.**
   http://www.emergencymed.arizona.edu/aemrc/paramedic.html

5. **California Physicians Medical Group.**
   http://www.cep.com/

6. **Clinical Evidence**. Straight from BMJ.
   http://www.clinicalevidence.com/ceweb/conditions/index.jsp

7. **David Baldwin's Trauma Pages.**
   http://www.trauma-pages.com/

8. **Dermatlas**. An amazing visual aid.
   http://dermatlas.med.jhmi.edu/derm/

9. **Drug Doses in Emergency Medicine**. Like a bible to physicians.
   http://www.priory.co.uk/emerg.htm

10. **ECG Learning Center.** Got-to-have site!
    http://library.med.utah.edu/kw/ecg/

11. **Emergency First Aid.** Very simple but informative.
    http://www.healthy.net/scr/MainLinks.asp?Id=170

12. **Emergency Medicine Online**. Find something interesting.
    http://www.emed.org/

13. **Emergency Medicine Ultrasound**. Bread and butter for ER doctors.
    http://emultrasound.com/

14. **Emergency Medicine Web Portal**. Lots of useful links.
    http://www.mednets.com/index.cfm/fuseaction/articles_emergency_
    medicine_databases_search_engines_semerg

15. **e-Residency.** Online residency management system.
    http://www.eresidency.net/

16. **Emergency Room Stat**. An EM heaven.
    http://www.erstat.com/

17. **Evidence Based Med Toolkit.**
    http://www.med.ualberta.ca/ebm/ebm.htm

18. **Fire and EMS Information Network.**
    http://cms.firehouse.com/content/fhnet/

19. **Institute for Emergency Medical Education.**
    http://www.ifeme.com/about.php

20. **Interactive Cyber Rounds.**
    http://www.cyberounds.com/

21. **International EMS.** Beyond borders.
    http://www.international-ems.com/forum/

22. **Injury-Related Web sites/CDC.**
    http://www.cdc.gov/ncipc/injweb/websites.htm

23. **Emergency Medicine 911**. A paramedics special.
    http://www.emergency-med.com/

24. **Medic Alert**. Nonprofit health care informatics organization.
    http://www.medicalert.org/home/Homegradient.aspx

25. **Merginet.** A virtual reading room of EMS information.
    http://www.merginet.com/

26. **Mobile PDR.**
    http://www.pdr.net/login/Login.aspx

27. **Prehospital Care Research Forum**. Promotion, education, and dissemination of prehospital research.
    http://www.pcrf.mednet.ucla.edu/

28. **Rallye Rejviz**. Czech Republic EMS.
    http://www.rallye-rejviz.cz/

29. **Traumatic Brain Injuries.** Pretty much everything you need to know.
    http://www.aitken.org/

30. **Trauma X-Ray Collection.** Images of key trauma x-rays.
    http://www.swsahs.nsw.gov.au/livtrauma/education/xray.asp

31. **Concussion Checklist. Nice outline.**
    http://www.health.state.ok.us/program/injury/updates/ concussion.html

32. **Pediatric Emergency Resuscitation Guide.**
    http://circ.ahajournals.org/cgi/content/full/95/8/2185

33. **PainEDU.org.** Series of different courses for health care practitioners.
    http://www.painedu.org/course.asp

34. **Medical Spanish-English Translator Form.**
http://www.erworld.com/medspan.htm

35. **Emergency Medicine Litigation Analysts**. A complete start-to-finish litigation support.
http://www.erexperts.com/index.htm

36. **ER 365**. A free emergency medicine job site.
http://www.er365.com/

37. **Emergency Medicine Interest Group.** To connect students with faculty advisers.
http://medschool.ucsf.edu/medstudents/StudLife/orgs/emig/index.asp

38. **Emergency Medicine Network (EMNet).**
http://www.emnet-usa.org/emnet_details.htm

39. **Regional Emergency Medical Services Council of New York City.**
http://www.nycremsco.org/protocols/remsco.html

40. **Medgadget**. Internet resource for emergent medical technologies.
http://medgadget.com/archives/emergency_medicine/

41. **BUBL LINK**. Catalogue of Internet emergency medicine resources in UK.
http://bubl.ac.uk/Link/e/emergencymedicine.htm

42. **Medical Corps's Combat Medicine**. A course for those who really want it.
http://www.medicalcorps.org/

43. **Emergency Medicine Experts Online.** Satisfaction guarantee.
http://www.kasamba.com/experts/health-medicine/emergency-medicine

44. **Emergency Multilingual Phrasebook**. Great download opportunity.
http://www.dh.gov.uk/assetRoot/04/07/32/82/04073282.pdf

45. **AEP LINKS**. This is proudly presented by Association of Emergency Physicia4ns.
   http://www.aep.org/links.asp

46. **Emergency Medicine on CD-ROM**. Pretty much everything in the world of EM.
   http://www.medicalamazon.com/emergency-medicine.html

47. **MedLink Neurology**. The most comprehensive resource for neurology.
   www.medlink.com/medlinkcontent.asp

12. Emergency Department Documentation Systems

1. **Emergisoft ED**. Complete emergency department information system.
    http://www.emergisoft.com/

2. **ePowerDoc.** ED Documentation.
    http://www.epowerdoc.com/

3. **E/Map System/Lynx Medical Systems.**
    http://www.lynxmed.com/

4. **Seacrest Medical Review**. Provides technical expertise, inspiration, and guidance.
    http://www.mbhc.com/src.htm

5. **T-System**. Implementing powerful template charting solutions.
    http://www.tsystem.com/

6. **Vital Works.** A leader in radiology and medical image and information management solutions.
    http://www.amicas.com/

7. **X-Press Charts.** Pioneered in emergency medicine documentation.
    http://www.xpresscharts.com/

8. **Emergency Medicine Coding.** Here comes an expert.
    http://www.codingnetwork.com/emergency-medicine-coding.html

9. **CBIZ.** Provides comprehensive medical billing coder services.
    http://www.cbiz.com/page.asp?pid=3211

13. Emergency Physicians Practice Resources

1. **California Emergency Physicians (MedAmerica).** Offers a comprehensive menu of proven practice management services.
    http://www.medamerica.com/

2. **CompHealth.** Providers of health care staffing and recruiting services.
    http://www.comphealth.com/

3. **ED Care's Management.** Health care services management company.
    http://www.edcaremgt.com/

4. **EmCare.** Leading provider of emergency care.
    http://www.emcare.com/DesktopDefault.aspx

5. **EMedForum.** The best emergency medicine forum online!
    http://www.emedforum.com/index.php

6. **Emergency Consultants, Inc.** Physician recruiting, staffing, and management.
    http://www.eci-med.com/

7. **Emergency Medical Associates (EMA).**
    http://www.ema-ed.com/

8. **Emergency Medical Care (EMC).**
    http://www.emcphysicians.com/

9. **Emergency Medicine Consultants, Ltd.**
    http://www.emdocs.com/

10. **Emergency Medicine Physicians, Ltd.**
    http://www.emp.com/

11. **Emergency Practice Associates**. Offers a comprehensive program of physician services.
    http://www.epamidwest.com/

12. **Hayman Daugherty Associates, Inc.**
    http://www.haymandaugherty.com/

13. **Linde Healthcare**. Specializes in the recruitment of locum tenens physicians.
    http://www.lindehc.com/

14. **The NES Healthcare Group**. Providing high quality, cost-efficient services.
    http://www.neshold.com/

15. **Phoenix Physicians**. Experience, stability, service, and innovation.
    http://www.phoenixphysicians.com/

16. **Physicians Staffing Resources**. Emergency medicine business experts.
    http://www.psrinc.net/

17. **Premier Health Care Services**. Provide the highest quality of health care.
    http://www.premierhcs.net/

18. **Southwest Medical Associates, Inc.**
    http://www.swmed.com/

19. **Sheridan Emergency Physicians**. Most experienced outsourcing provider for emergency medicine.
    http://www.sheridanhealthcare.com/main/index.html

20. **The Schumacher Group**. Adding value to our clients' emergency departments.
    http://www.tsged.com/

21. **Sterling Healthcare**. A national leader in the provisioning of clinical contract management service.
    http://www.sterlinghealthcare.com/new/

22. **Team Health**. Provides emergency department administrative and staffing services.
    http://www.teamhealth.com/

23. **United Emergency Services, Inc. (UES)**. Physician staffing company.
    http://www.unitedemergency.com/

24. **Valley Emergency Physicians Medical Group (VEP)**. Provides emergency medicine and primary care physician services.
    http://www.valleyemergency.com/

25. **Weatherby Locums**. Provides freedom and flexibility for locum tenens.
    http://www.weatherbylocums.com/index.html

26. **PracticeLink® Physician Emergency Medicine Jobs**. A very comprehensive list.
    http://www.practicelink.com/jobs/Physician/Emergency_Medicine/

27. **Emergency Medicine Job Search**. Straight from Emed mag.
    http://careers.emedmag.com/index.cfm

14. Emergency Medicine Organizations (North America)

1. American College of Emergency Physicians.
    http://www.acep.org/webportal

2. Society for Academic Emergency Medicine.
    http://www.saem.org/

3. Association of Emergency Physicians.
    http://www.aep.org/

4. American Board of Emergency Physicians.
    http://www.abem.org/public

5. American Academy of Emergency Medicine.
    http://www.aaem.org/

6. The American College of Osteopathic Emergency Physicians (ACOEP).
    http://www.acoep.org/

7. American Academy of Pediatrics.
    http://www.aap.org/

8. American Pediatric Society.
    http://www.aps-spr.org/

9. Canadian Association of Emergency Physicians.
    http://www.caep.ca/

10. **The Council of Emergency Medicine Residency Directors (CORD).**
    A scientific and educational organization.
    http://www.cordem.org/

11. **Emergency Medicine Residents Association.**
    http://www.emra.org/

12. **National Association of EMS Physicians.**
    http://www.naemsp.org/

13. **Quebec Emergency Medicine Association.**
    http://www.urgenet.qc.ca/

14. **The Massachusetts College of Emergency Physicians.**
    http://www.macep.org/index.htm

15. **The Society of Emergency Medicine Physician Assistants (SEMPA)**
    http://www.sempa.org/

16. **American Medical Association (AMA).** Helping doctors help patients.
    http://www.ama-assn.org/

17. **Medical Society of the State of New York (MSSNY).**
    http://www.mssny.org/

18. **National Emergency Medicine Association.**
    http://www.nemahealth.org/

19. **Emergency Medicine Interest Resource.**
    http://southmed.usouthal.edu/emig/resources.html

20. **The Emergency Department Practice Management Association (EDPMA)**
    http://www.edpma.com/i4a/pages/index.cfm?pageid=1

21. **American Burn Association.**
    http://www.ameriburn.org/

22. **Emergency Medicine Student Association (EMSA).** Strives to educate current medical students.
http://www.med.fsu.edu/students/EMSA/default.asp

23. **The Institute for Emergency Medical Education (IEME).**
http://www.ifeme.com/about.php

24. **Federal Emergency Management Agency (FEMA).**
http://www.fema.gov/index.shtm

25. **National Emergency Management Association (NEMA).**
http://www.nemaweb.org/index.cfm

26. **National Registry of Emergency Medical Technicians (NREMT).**
http://www.nremt.org/about/nremt_news.asp

27. **American Trauma Society.**
http://www.amtrauma.org/

28. **The American Association for the Surgery of Trauma.**
http://www.aast.org/

29. **Air Medical Physician Association.**
http://www.ampa.org/

30. **Emergency Care Research Institute.** Health care research and quality.
http://www.ecri.org/

31. **Emergency Medicine Cardiac Research Education Group.** An international research and education network.
http://www.emcreg.org/index.html

32. **The American Academy of Urgent Care Medicine (AAUCM).**
http://www.aaucm.org/

15. International Emergency Medicine Organizations

1. Australasian College for Emergency Medicine.
    http://www.acem.org.au/home.aspx?docID=1

2. Association for Emergency Medicine in France.
    http://www.amuhf.com/

3. Asian Society for Emergency Medicine.
    http://www.asem.org.sg/

4. European Society for Emergency Medicine.
    http://www.eusem.org/

5. British Association for Accident and EM.
    http://www.emergencymed.org.uk/BAEM

6. Costa Rica Association of Emergency Medicine.
    http://http://www.cne.go.cr/

7. Hong Kong College of Emergency Medicine.
    http://www.hkam.org.hk/colleges/em.htm

8. International Emergency Medicine Rotations Database.
    http://www.ed.bmc.org/iem/search.cfm

9. The Society for Emergency Medicine in Taiwan.
    http://www.sem.org.tw/

10. Society for Emergency Medicine in Singapore.
     http://www.semsonline.org/

11. The Spanish Society for Emergency Medicine.
     http://www.semes.org/

12. The Spanish Society for Pediatric Emergencies.
     http://www.seup.org/seup/index.html

13. Bahrain Emergentologist Association.
     http://www.bemasso.org/

14. The Web site of Emergency Medicine in Belgium.
     http://www.emerbel.org/default.htm

15. Estonian Society of Emergency Medicine.
     http://www.kiirabi.ee/

16. Portugal Institute of National Emergency Medicine.
     http://www.inem.pt/

17. The Irish Association for Emergency Medicine.
     http://www.iaem.ie/

18. The Israeli Society of Emergency Medicine.
     http://isrjem.org/

19. The Korean Society of Emergency Medicine.
     http://www.emergency.or.kr/

20. Lithuanian Society for Emergency Medicine.
     http://www.kmu.lt/emed

21. The Netherlands Association for Emergency Physicians.
     http://www.nvsha.nl/home.asp

22. Pan-Arab Society of Trauma & Emergency Medicine.
     http://www.hmc.org.qa/pastem/home.htm

23. Polish Society for Emergency Medicine.
http://www.medycynaratunkowa.com.pl

24. Slovenian Societies for Emergency Medicine.
http://www.ssem-society.si

25. The Argentinean Society for Emergency Medicine.
http://www.emergencias.org/ID1/00001.htm

26. Italian Society of Emergency Medicine.
http://www.simeu.it/file.php?file=dir&sez=articoli&id=15&ses=15

27. The Society for Emergency Medicine India.
http://www.smfhospital.org/semisite/index.htm

28. Society for Emergency Medicine Singapore.
http://www.semsonline.org/

29. Spanish Society for Urgent & Emergency Medicine.
http://www.semes.org/

30. Swedish Society for Emergency Medicine, SweSEM.
http://www.swesem.org/

31. Emergency Medicine Association of Turkey.
http://www.tatd.org.tr/

32. The Czech Society of Emergency and Disaster Medicine.
http://www.urgmed.cz/

33. The Dutch Society of Emergency Medicine.
http://www.nvsha.nl/

34. Pediatric Emergency Medicine Israel (PEMI).
http://health.groups.yahoo.com/group/PEMI/

35. Societa Italiana di Medicina di Emergenza e Urgenza Pediatrica
(SIMEUP).
http://www.simeup.com/

36. Emergency Medicine Researchers International.
    http://www.dwwalsh.com/

37. European Society for Emergency Medicine.
    http://www.diesis.com/eusem/aims.htm

38. World Association for Disaster and Emergency Medicine.
    http://wadem.medicine.wisc.edu/

16. Emergency Medicine Nurses Resources

1. **Emergency Nurses Association.**
    http://www.ena.org/

2. **Board of Certification in Emergency Nursing.**
    http://www.ena.org/bcen/cen/

3. **Forensic Nurses Association.**
    http://www.forensicnurse.org/

4. **Journal of Emergency Nursing.**
    http://journals.elsevierhealth.com/periodicals/ymen

5. **Safe Kids Worldwide.**
    http://www.safekids.org/

6. **The Society of Trauma Nurses.**
    http://www.traumanursesoc.org/

7. **The Entire World of Emergency Nursing.**
    http://enw.org/Basic.htm

8. **New York Emergency Room RN.**
    http://www.nyerrn.com/

9. **American Association of Critical Care Nurses.**
    http://www.aacn.org/

10. **Air & Surface Transport Nurses Association.**
    http://www.astna.org/

11. **Virtual Nurse.** Nursing reference portal.
    http://www.virtualnurse.com/

12. **ImpactEDNurses.com**. You've got to read this one!
    http://impactednurse.com/

17. Emergency Medical Services

1. National Association of EMS Physicians.
    http://www.naemsp.org/

2. The Internet Gateway for EMS Professionals.
    http://www.mhf.net/Default.asp

3. Nassau Regional EMS Council.
    http://www.nassauems.com/

4. Paramedic Program at Stony Brook.
    http://www.mic.ki.se/Nursing.html

5. Emergency Medical Technician Paramedic: National Standard
    Curriculum.
    http://www.nhtsa.dot.gov/people/injury/ems/EMT-P/index.html

6. EMS House. Premier site for EMS responders, instructors, and students.
    http://www.defrance.org/

7. Regional Emergency Medical Services Council of New York City.
    http://www.nycremsco.org/

8. Wilderness EMS Institute.
    http://www.wemsi.org/

9. Emergency Medical Service for Children.
    http://www.ems-c.org/

10. **Pediatric EMS**. Lots of resources on the site.
    http://www.pemdatabase.org/ems.html

11. **Trauma Team EMS Protocols.** Extensive resource for the EMS protocols.
    **http://www.ssgfx.com/CP2020/medtech/procedures/protocols.
    htm#quick_ref**

12. **SWAT Doctors.** Health care providers who have taken the initiative,
    time, and training to practice tactical emergency medicine.
    http://www.swatdoctor.com/pages/1/index.htm

13. **Radford University Emergency Medical Services.**
    http://www.runet.edu/~ruems

14. **The Brandies Emergency Medical Corps.**
    http://www.unet.brandeis.edu/~bemco

15. **Pediatric Education for Prehospital Professionals**. Great resource for EMS.
    http://www.peppsite.com/

16. **The Electronic Newsletter of Prehospital Cardiac Care.** Latest
    information on prehospital cardiac care.
    http://www.mhf.net/Threshold

17. **EMS Dedicated Medical Books.**
    **http://www.emergencybookstore.com/ home_store.aspx?StoreCod
    e=EMS%20Books**

18. **The Ultimate EMS Resource. Great site!**
    http://www.merginet.com/

19. **A leadership guide to EMS**. Distributed by the U.S. Department of
    Transportation.
    **http://www.nhtsa.dot.gov/people/injury/ems/leaderguide/index.
    html**

20. **EMS Medical Product. An online catalog.**
    http://www.eventmedical.com/

21. **Jems.com**. EMS online resource.
    http://www.jems.com/

22. **American Ambulance Association.**
    http://www.the-aaa.org/

23. **International Trauma Life support.**
    http://www.itrauma.org/

24. **The Commission on Accreditation of Ambulance Services (CAAS).**
    http://www.caas.org/

25. **Best Practices in EMS.**
    http://www.emsbest.com/

26. **EMS Village**. Great source of information.
    http://www.emsvillage.com/

27. **Flightweb**. Air medical service.
    http://www.flightweb.com/index.php

28. **Medic Planet.** Great source of information for the health professional.
    http://www.medicplanet.com/

29. **Less Stress Instructional Services**. Basic resuscitation tools.
    http://www.lessstress.com/

30. **Pre-Hospital Trauma Life Support**. A resource and tool for PHTLS providers.
    http://www.naemt.org/PHTLS/

31. **The FIREMedic**. If you like fires!
    http://www.firemedic.com/

32. **Emergency Medical Services Corporation.**
    http://www.emsc.net/

33. **Geriatric Education for Emergency Medical Services.**
    http://www.gemssite.com/

34. **National Association of EMTs.**
    http://www.naemt.org/

35. **The Association of Air Medical Services (AAMS).**
    http://www.aams.org/aboutaams.html

36. **National EMS Memorial Service.**
    http://nemsms.org/

37. **JEMSprepare.** Unparalleled continuing education program for EMS personnel.
    http://www.mywebce.com/index.asp?a=Home

38. **Emergency Medical Services.** Potpourri of EMS.
    http://www.skyaid.org/Skyaid%20Org/Medical/EMS.htm

39. **American Ambulance Association.**
    http://www.the-aaa.org/

40. **National EMS Pilots Association (NEMSPA).**
    http://www.nemspa.org/index2.php

41. **Advanced Rescue Technology.** Serving first responders.
    http://www.advancedrt.com/

18. International Emergency Medicine

1. **Practice Medicine in Developing World.**
    http://www.remotemedicine.org/

2. **International Emergency Medicine Rotations Database.**
    http://www.ed.bmc.org/iem/search.cfm

3. **International Emergency Medicine (Current Activities)**. Great site
    for those who are really interested.
    http://www.usc.edu/schools/medicine/departments/emergency_
    medicine/international/Pages/current_activities.html

4. **International Emergency Medicine Disaster Specialists.**
    http://www.iemds.com/

5. **The Institute for International Emergency Medicine and Health
    (IEMH)**. Dedicated to developing improvements in emergency health care.
    http://www.iemh.org/

6. **International Medical Corps**. Global humanitarian nonprofit
    organization.
    http://www.imcworldwide.org/about.shtml

7. **Doctors without Borders**. Delivers emergency aid to people affected.
    http://www.dwb.org/

8. **International Committee of the Red Cross**
    http://www.icrc.org/

9. **Emergency Medicine Researchers International.** A service of Walsh & Walsh.
   http://www.dwwalsh.com/

10. **The International School of Tactical Medicine.**
    http://www.tacticalmedicine.com/

11. **INTERNATIONAL EMERGENCY MEDICINE LITERATURE. EMRA SPECIAL.**
    http://www.emra.org/Index.cfm?FuseAction=Page&PageID=1002028

12. **UCLA Center for Emergency Medicine.**
    http://www.ciem.ucla.edu/

13. **International Emergency Medicine of Australia.**
    http://www.acem.org.au/infocentre.aspx?docId=55

14. **Emergency Medicine Cardiac Research and Education Group International.**
    http://www.emcreg.org/

15. **The ArabMedicare.com.** Emergency Medicine Center.
    http://www.arabmedicare.com/emergency.htm

16. **Medicine International.** More facts about Medicine International.
    http://www.medicineinternational.org/morefacts.html

17. **Salient Training in Emergency Medicine International (STEMI).**
    http://www.stemi.com.au/

18. **International Clinical Trials in Trauma/Emergency Medicine.**
    http://www.centerwatch.com/cwworld/world_area20.html

19. **Doctors of the World (USA).** International health and human rights organization.
    http://www.doctorsoftheworld.org/

20. **Healing Hands International.** Serves to save lives and relieve suffering.
    http://www.hhi.org/about-us.php

19. Journals

1. **Academic Emergency Medicine.**
   http://www.aemj.org/

2. **Annals of Emergency Medicine**. You might have to go through the Elsevier Publishing.
   http://www.annemergmed.com/

3. **The American Journal of Emergency Medicine.**
   http://www.sciencedirect.com/

4. **Academic Medicine**. Peer-reviewed monthly.
   http://www.academicmedicine.org/

5. **American Journal of Respiratory and Critical Care.**
   http://intl-ajrccm.atsjournals.org/

6. **British Medical Journal Online.**
   http://www.bmj.com/

7. **Canadian Journal of Emergency Medicine.**
   http://www.caep.ca/

8. **Canadian Medical Association Journal.**
   http://www.cmaj.ca/

9. **Clinical Pediatric Emergency Medicine**. You go through Science Direct.
   http://www.sciencedirect.com/

10. **Critical Care Clinic**. Go through Elsevier Publishing.
    http://www.journals.elsevierhealth.com/home

11. **Emergency Medical Abstracts Online.**
    http://www.ccme.org/

12. **Emergency Medicine Clinic of North America**. One of my favorites.
    http://www.journals.elsevierhealth.com/home

13. **Emergency Medicine Magazine.**
    http://www.emedmag.com/

14. **Emergency Medicine News.**
    http://www.EM-NEWS.com/

15. **Emergency Medicine Journal.**
    http://http://emj.bmjjournals.com/

16. **Elsevier Science Direct**. Major publishing company for EM.
    http://www.elsevier.com/

17. **The Medical Journal of Australia (EMMA).**
    http://www.mja.com.au/

18. **The European Journal of Emergency Medicine.**
    http://www.euro-emergencymed.com/pt/re/ejem/home.htm

19. **Emergency Medicine Journal Watch.**
    http://emergency-medicine.jwatch.org/

20. **Emergency Radiology.**
    http://www.springerlink.com/content/1438-1435/

21. **European Journal of Trauma.**
    http://www.springerlink.com/content/1615-3146/

22. **Hospital Physician**. Includes five journals.
    http://www.turner-white.com/

23. Injury.
    http://www.elsevier.com/wps/find/journaldescription.cws_home/
    30428/description#description

24. International Journal of Mass Emergencies and Disasters.
    http://www.usc.edu/schools/sppd/ijmed/

25. Internet Journal of Emergency and Intensive Care Medicine.
    http://www.ispub.com/ostia/index.php?xmlFilePath=journals/
    ijeicm/front.xml

26. Internet Journal of Rescue and Disaster Medicine.
    http://www.ispub.com/ostia/index.php?xmlFilePath=journals/
    ijrdm/front.xml

27. The Journal of American Medical Association.
    http://www.jama.ama-assn.org

28. A Journal of Clinical Emergency Medicine.
    http://www.medical-library.org/j_er.htm

29. The Journal of Emergency Medicine. Truly great source, great cases.
    http://www.elsevier.com/wps/find/journaldescription.cws_
    home/525473/description#description

30. Journal of Intensive Care Medicine.
    http://jic.sagepub.com/

31. Journal of the American Medical Informatics Association.
    http://www.jamia.org/

32. Journal of Accidents & Emergency Medicine (Worldcat Libraries).
    http://www.worldcatlibraries.org/oclc/30325995&referer=brief_
    results

33. Journal of Trauma.
    http://www.jtrauma.com/

34. **Middle East Journal of Emergency Medicine.**
http://www.hmc.org.qa/hmcnewsite/

35. **Morbidity and Mortality Weekly Reports.**
http://www.cdc.gov/mmwr

36. **Pediatric Emergency Care.**
http://www.pec-online.com/

37. **Practical Summaries in Acute Care.**
http://www.ahcpub.com/

38. **Resident & Staff Physician.**
http://www.residentandstaff.com/

39. **Resuscitation.**
http://www.elsevier.com/wps/find/journaldescription.cws_
home/505959/description#description

40. **Postgraduate Medicine Online.**
http://www.postgradmed.com/

41. **Free Medical Journals**. A got-to-see site!
http://www.freemedicaljournals.com/

42. **Shock.**
http://www.shocksocieties.org/international/shockjournal/

43. **The New England Journal of Medicine.**
http://www.nejm.org/

44. **Pediatric Emergency Medicine Reports.**
http://www.ahcpub.com/archive/

45. **Israeli Journal of Emergency Medicine.**
http://isrjem.org/

46. **Emergency Medicine Australasia.**
http://www.blackwellpublishing.com/journal.asp?ref=1742-6731&site=1

47. **Resuscitation**. Read your brain off.
http://www.sciencedirect.com/

48. **The Internet Journal of Emergency and Intensive Care Medicine.** Great online source.
http://www.ispub.com/ostia/index.php?xmlFilePath=journals/ijeicm/ front.xml

49. **The Lancet Journals.**
http://www.thelancet.com/

50. **The Free Medical Journals.** Great list of various medical journals.
http://www.freemedicaljournals.com/

51. **Year Book of Emergency Medicine.**
http://www.us.elsevierhealth.com/product.jsp?isbn=02717964

52. **Accident & Emergency Nursing.**
http://www.harcourt-international.com/journals/aaen/

53. **Advances in Skin & Wound Care.**
http://www.aswcjournal.com/

54. **Air Medical Journal.**
http://journals.elsevierhealth.com/periodicals/ymam/

55. **American Journal of Critical Care.**
http://ajcc.aacnjournals.org/

56. **Journal of the International Society for Burn Injuries.**
http://www.chinaburn.net/zyzy/ShowArticle.asp?ArticleID=124

57. **Clinical Pediatric Emergency Medicine.**
http://www.us.elsevierhealth.com/product.jsp?isbn=15228401

58. **Welcome to Critical Care**. The online journal for intensivists.
http://ccforum.com/

59. **Critical Care Medicine.**
http://www.ccmjournal.com/

60. **Critical Care Nursing Clinics of North America.**
http://www.us.elsevierhealth.com/product.jsp?isbn=08995885

61. **Current Opinion in Critical Care.**
http://www.co-criticalcare.com/

62. **Disaster Management and Response.**
http://www.disastermgmt.com/

63. **Emergency Medical Abstracts.**
http://prod2.ccme.org/ema/

64. **Emergency Nurse.**
http://www.nursing-standard.co.uk/emergencynurse/index.asp

65. **The EMS Insider.**
http://www.jems.com/emsinsider/

66. **Intensive Care Medicine.**
http://www.springerlink.com/content/1432-1238/

67. **International Wound Journal (IWJ).**
http://www.blackwellpublishing.com/journal.asp?ref=1742-4801&site=1

68. **The Med Connect**. An online journal for health professional.
http://www.medconnect.com/

69. **Journal of Burn Care & Research.**
http://www.burncarerehab.com/

70. **Journal of Cardiac Failure.**
http://journals.elsevierhealth.com/periodicals/yjcaf

71. **The Journal of Critical Care.**
    http://journals.elsevierhealth.com/periodicals/yjcrc

72. **A Journal of Clinical Emergency Medicine.**
    http://www.ccspublishing.com/j_er.htm

73. **Neurocritical Care.**
    http://humanapress.com/

74. **Nursing in Critical Care.**
    http://www.blackwellpublishing.com/journal.asp?ref=1362-1017

75. **Pediatric Critical Care Medicine.**
    http://www.pccmjournal.com/

76. **Prehospital Emergency Care.**
    http://www.tandf.co.uk/journals/titles/10903127.asp

77. **Seminars in Respiratory and Critical Care Medicine.**
    http://www.thieme.com/SID1993373986839/journals/pubid1393
    790216.html

78. **World Wide Wound. The premier online resource for dressing materials and practical wound management information.**
    http://www.worldwidewounds.com/

79. **Wound Repair and Regeneration.**
    http://www.blackwellpublishing.com/journal.asp?ref=1067-
    1927&site=1

20. Pediatric Emergency Medicine

1. **PALS**. The pediatric emergency medicine resource.
    http://www.aplsonline.com/

2. **Pediatric Emergency Medicine Database**. Absolutely a must-read!
    http://www.pemdatabase.org/

3. **Pediatric research in Emergency Therapeutics**. Very nice site with
    lots of information.
    http://www.pretx.org/

4. **Pediatric Emergency Medicine practical tools**. All you need to have!
    http://www.pemdatabase.org/pemtools.html

5. **PEDIATRICS Subspecialty Collections. In-depth, up-to-date pediatrics.**
    http://pediatrics.aappublications.org/collections

6. **The Center for Pediatric Emergency Medicine**. Well, home for PEM.
    http://www.cpem.org

7. **PediatricEducation.org.** Pediatric digital library and learning resources.
    http://www.pediatriceducation.org/

8. **Pediatric ECG of the Week**. A weekly ECG to challenge those learning
    and reading pediatric ECGs.
    http://www.paedcard.com/

9. **Emergency Medical Services for Children**. Extensive EMS-based site.
    http://www.ems-c.org/

10. **Emergency Pediatrics (Canadian Paediatric Society).**
http://www.cps.ca/english/publications/EmergPaediatrics.htm

11. **American Academy of Pediatrics.** Check the section of emergency medicine.
http://www.aap.org/sections/PEM

12. **Virtual Children's Hospital**. Great resource for everyone.
http://www.virtualpediatrichospital.org/

13. **Pediatric Database** online resource for pediatric critical care.
http://utenti.unife.it/giampaolo.garani/Trauma/Trauma-Ped/Peds
CCM%20File%20Cabinet.htm

14. **Electronic Article: Drugs for Pediatric Emergencies**. A must-read.
http://pediatrics.aappublications.org/cgi/content/full/101/1/e13

15. **PedsCCM: The Pediatric Critical Care Web site.**
http://pedsccm.org/

16. **Pediatric Medicine Sites**. Great selection from Yahoo!
http://dir.yahoo.com/Health/medicine/pediatrics/

17. **An Imaging Encyclopedia of Pediatric Disease.** Enormous amount of great information.
http://www.virtualpediatrichospital.org/providers/PAP/PAPHome.shtml

18. **Pediatric Emergency Medicine Practice**. You have to know this one!
http://ebmedpractice.net/

19. **Selected topics in Pediatrics**. Various neonatal and pediatric files in .doc and text format.
http://www.geocities.com/SouthBeach/Pointe/5375/Dailybread/Medical/Medical.html

20. **Radiology Cases in Pediatric Emergency Medicine.**
http://www.netmedicine.com/pediatric/v1/vol1.htm

21. **Pediatric-emergency.com.**
http://pediatric-emergency.com/

21. Medical Informatics and Devices

Palm Medical Resources

1. **Listing of software for Palms.** A must-have site!
    http://umed.med.utah.edu/pda/index.cfm

2. **PalmGear.Com.** One of the most comprehensive sites for general *palm organizer* tools.
    http://www.palmgear.com/

3. **Ectopic Brain.** A very nice site with medical news.
    http://pbrain.hypermart.net/index.html

4. **Handheldmed.** Connect with the future of medicine today. The latest in medical palm software.
    http://www.handheldmed.com/Site.New/Pages.php?p=home

5. **Skyscape**. Very impressive medical software but pricey.
    http://www.skyscape.com/index/home.aspx

6. **Medical Eponyms for the Palm.**
    http://eponyms.net/eponyms.htm

7. **Medical iSilo Depot**. Medical references for the doctor on the go.
    http://www.meistermed.com/isilodepot/isilo_depot_index_subj.htm

8. **Handheld recommendations from Dalhousie University**. Great software list.
    http://handheld.medicine.dal.ca/software/textbook.htm

9. **MemoWare.** Large searchable collections of medical palm tool applications
   http://www.memoware.com/

10. **The Dog Patch—Pilot First Aid Page.** Variety of files for the 3Com
    Palm Pilot.
    http://www.dogpatch.org/firstaid.html

11. **Physik's PalmPilot Pages.** Application with list of 850 memory aids in
    thirteen categories.
    http://www.access-company.com/support/links/index.html

12. **Kruzlifix's Download Page.** Graphic illustration of ACL reconstruction.
    http://www.staehelin.ch/download/download.html

13. **Selected topics in Pediatrics.** Various neonatal and pediatric files in
    .doc and text format.
    http://www.geocities.com/SouthBeach/Pointe/5375/Dailybread/
    Medical/Medical.html

14. **Stat ICD-9 coder.** Great software.
    http://statcode.hypermart.net/

15. **Electronic Medical Record Software.**
    http://www.a4healthsystems.com/

16. **National Center for Emergency Medicine Informatics.** Absolutely
    the best site!
    http://ncemi.org/

17. **Medscientist Software.** Educational software for medical professionals.
    http://www.madsci.com/

18. **HealthMatics® ED.** The most comprehensive Emergency Department
    Information System (EDIS).
    http://www.a4healthsystems.com/edis

19. **Healthy Palmpilot.** Must-see site on health care resource index.
    http://www.healthypalmpilot.com/

20. **PdaMD.com**. Simply the best!
    http://www.pdamd.com/vertical/home.xml

21. **MobileMICROMEDEX**. For Palm OS and Pocket PC.
    http://www.micromedex.com/products/clinicalxpert/

22. **Medical Piloteer.** Dedicated to linking sites that provide medical and/or health care resources for handheld devices.
    http://w.webring.com/hub?ring=medpilot

23. **MedGadget**. A journal of emerging medical technologies.
    http://www.medgadget.com/

24. **Emergency Medicine Constellation**. All-in-one emergency medicine solution.
    http://www.skyscape.com/EStore/ProductDetail.aspx?ProductID =1045

22. NBC Terrorism

1. **Anthrax from Armed Forces**. Information about the pathogenesis and imaging of inhalational anthrax.
    http://anthrax.radpath.org/

2. **Armed Forces Radiobiology Institute.**
    http://www.afrri.usuhs.mil/

3. **ATRSD (Managing Hazardous Material Incidents).**
    http://www.atsdr.cdc.gov/mhmi.html

4. **Bioterrorism and Emerging Infections**. Regularly updated resource information and free online continuing education.
    http://www.bioterrorism.uab.edu/

5. **Bioterrorism Agents/Diseases.** A must-read site.
    http://www.bt.cdc.gov/Agent/Agentlist.asp

6. **CDC (Emergency Preparedness and Response).**
    http://www.bt.cdc.gov/

7. **Hazmat for Healthcare**. Course and training programs for hospitals.
    http://hazmatforhealthcare.org/index.cfm?section=1

8. **Medical Management of Biological Casualties Handbook**. Got to read!
    http://library.advanced.org/21659/links.html

9. **Radiation Emergency Assistant Center**. The medical management of radiation accidents.
http://www.orau.gov/reacts

10. **The Metro New York Disaster Medical Assistance Team**. Designed to provide emergency medical care during a disaster or other event.
http://www.dmatny2.org/

11. **Investigation of Bioterrorism.** Related to anthrax.
http://www.cdc.gov/mmwr/preview/mmwrhtml/mm5043a1.htm

12. **Nuclear, Biological, and Chemical Medical Web page**. Great site.
http://www.geocities.com/Pentagon/Quarters/4389/

13. **National Disaster Medical System (NDMS).**
http://ndms.dhhs.gov/

14. **Treatments of Radionuclide Contamination.**
http://www.bordeninstitute.army.mil/nuclearwarfare/chapter4/chapter4.pdf

15. **National Homeland Security Knowledgebase**. Got to read.
http://www.nationalhomelandsecurityknowledgebase.com/

23. Pharmaceuticals

1. **Welcome to RXMed.** The Web site for physicians and patients. A great source of information.
   http://www.rxmed.com/

2. **Physician Desk References Online**. Got to have it.
   http://www.pdr.net/Home/Home.aspx

3. **Drug Information Center (Frequently Asked Questions).** Good site to use.
   http://www.uic.edu/pharmacy/services/di/di_faqs.htm

4. **Drug Shortage Pages**. From DEA offices.
   http://www.fda.gov/cder/drug/shortages/default.htm

5. **Antibiotic-Consult Online**. Your guide to antibiotic management on the Web.
   http://www.antibiotic-consult.com/

6. **Drug Shortage Resource Center-great information site.**
   http://www.ashp.org/s_ashp/resolved_shortages.asp?CID=1500&DID=1544&sort=0

7. **Rx Security. Supplier of counterfeit-resistant prescription pads.**
   http://www.rxsecurity.com/

8. **Medi-lexicon (formerly Pharma-Lexicon)**. Medical dictionary, pharmaceutical company search, and medical abbreviations.
   http://www.medilexicon.com/

9. **Welcome to Tarascon Publishing**. Ultimate drug information resource.
    http://www.tarascon.com/index.php

10. **RxList**. The Internet drug index.
    http://rxlist.com/

11. **Drug@FDA.** A catalog of FDA-approved drug products.
    http://www.accessdata.fda.gov/scripts/cder/drugsatfda/index.cfm

12. **Epocrates Reference Online**. Premium reference to clinicians.
    http://www2.epocrates.com/index.html

13. **Welcome to MyDrugRep.com**. Your around-the-clock resource for
    pharmaceuticals.
    http://www.mydrugrep.com/default.asp?bhcp=1

14. **The Renal Drug Book**. Providing dose guidelines for adult drug
    prescriptions in renal failure.
    http://www.renalnet.org/
    http://www.globalrph.com/renaldosing.htm (GlobalRPh.com.)

15. **Antimicrobial Agents and Chemotherapy**. Major forum exclusively
    devoted to antimicrobial, antiviral, antifungal, and antiparasitic agents.
    http://aac.asm.org/

24. Practice Guidelines in EM

1. **National Guideline Clearinghouse.**
    http://www.guideline.gov/

2. **Guidelines Advisory Committee.**
    http://www.gacguidelines.ca/

3. **ACEP Clinical Policies.**
    http://www.acep.org/webportal/PracticeResources/Clinical
    Policies/

4. **The CAEP Committee.** The Canadian EM guidelines.
    http://www.caep.ca/template.asp?id=37C951DE051A45979A9BD
    D0C5715C9FE

5. **Clinical Guidelines for Care of the Emergency Patient.**
    http://www.ed.bmc.org/emguidelines/guideem.html

6. **Primary Care Clinical Practice Guidelines.**
    http://medicine.ucsf.edu/resources/guidelines/index.html

25. Radiology and Images

I. Emergency Radiology

1. **Emergency Radiology Primer.** Nice way to start.
   http://www.uth.tmc.edu/radiology/test/er_primer/index.html

2. **CT in Head Trauma.** Tutorial to everything you need to know.
   http://www.radiology.co.uk/srs-x/tutors/cttrauma/tutor.htm

3. **Trauma.org.** Image bank.
   http://www.trauma.org/

4. **Emergency Body CT.** Speaks for itself.
   http://www.med-ed.virginia.edu/courses/rad/abdtrauma/

5. **Emergency Ultrasound.** You've got to have this site!
   http://www.med-ed.virginia.edu/courses/rad/edus/index.html

6. **Imaging Evaluation of the Cervical Spine.** Keep the C-collar handy.
   http://www.med-ed.virginia.edu/courses/rad/cspine/

7. **Introduction to Head CT.**
   http://www.med-ed.virginia.edu/courses/rad/headct/

8. **Skeletal Trauma Radiology.**
   http://www.med-ed.virginia.edu/courses/rad/ext/

II. Radiology Images and Cases.

1. **Radiology Web**. Great resource.
    http://www.radiologyweb.com/

2. **Emergency Radiology Primer**. Site designed for radiology residents but worthwhile to look.
    http://www.uth.tmc.edu/radiology/test/er_primer/index.html

3. **Radiology Teaching Cases from Harvard**. One of my favorite.
    http://brighamrad.harvard.edu/education/online/tcd/tcd.html

4. **UW Radiology Teaching File**. Quick cases.
    http://www.rad.washington.edu/quickcases

5. **An Imaging Encyclopedia of Pediatric Disease**. Enormous amount of great information.
    http://www.virtualpediatrichospital.org/providers/PAP/ PAPHome.shtml

6. **Radiology Cases in Pediatric Emergency Medicine and Acute Care**.
    http://www.netmedicine.com/pediatric/v1/vol1.htm

7. **My PACS.net**. Reference case manager.
    http://www.mypacs.net/repos/mpv3_repo/static/m/Home/

8. **Radiology Cases in Pediatric Emergency Medicine Online**. Great site.
    http://www.hawaii.edu/medicine/pediatrics/pemxray/pemxray.html

9. **Teaching Files from Bhatia**. Nice collection of images.
    http://www.mribhatia.com/teaching%20files.html

10. **Department of Radiology Teaching File**.
    http://www.rad.uab.edu:591/tf

11. **Imaging Cases of the Week**. Good selection of images.
    http://home.earthlink.net/%7Eradiologist/tf/index.htm

12. **UHRAD**. In-depth diagnostic radiology.
    http://www.uhrad.com/

13. **MedPix (Medical Images Database)**. Great site.
    http://rad.usuhs.mil/medpix/medpix.html?mode=my_medpix

14. **SVHRAD.com**. Teaching files from St. Vincent.
    http://www.svhrad.com/cases/index.php

15. **Neuroradiology**. Interesting cases.
    http://www.neurorad.ucsf.edu/case

16. **Michael Tobin**. Great database of imaging files.
    http://www.mikety.net

17. **Clinical Cases Query**. Over 3,700 images.
    http://www.med.univ-rennes1.fr/cerf/ico_an/INDEXAN.HTM

18. **Radiology Case Museum**. A site with lots of images.
    http://myweb.lsbu.ac.uk/dirt/museum/museum.html

19. **EMedicine Radiology**. Large selection of rare images.
    http://www.emedicine.com/radio/contents.htm

20. **Radiology Teaching File Guide**. Preparing for the board by using teaching cases on the Internet.
    http://ej.rsna.org/ej2/0071-98.fin/default.htm

21. **Radiology Files from Wayne State University**
    http://www.med.wayne.edu/diagRadiology/TF/TeachingFile.html

22. **Interesting Ultrasound Cases**. From UCSF.
    http://ultrasound.ucsf.edu/USCases.html

23. **Clinical Case Presentations**. Great teaching cases prepared by residents from DuPont Hospital (Orthopedics Division).
    http://gait.aidi.udel.edu/res695/homepage/pd_ortho/educate/clincase/clcasehp.htm

24. **The Pediatric Radiology-Pathology Web Page.** Great resource for imaging.
    www.uab.edu/pedradpath/index.html

25. **Radiology Web sites.** Everything you may need.
    http://www.healthline.com/search?q1=radiology+teaching+files&imuId=2801347

26. **Learning Radiology Online.** I love this site!
    http://www.learningradiology.com/index.htm

27. **Emergency Radiology Primer.**
    http://www.uth.tmc.edu/radiology/test/er_primer/index.html

28. **Radiology Imaging Info.** A radiology heaven.
    http://web.info.com/infocom.us2/search/web/radiology%20imaging?CMP=3073&itkw=radiology%20imaging

29. **Radiology Teaching File & Case Review and Teaching File Links.** An oral board for radiologist—amazing resource.
    http://www.theoralboard.com/teachinglinks.html

30. **RadiologyEducation.com.** A digital library of radiology education resources.
    http://www.radiologyeducation.com/

26. Residency Stuff

1. Emergency Medicine Residency Association (EMRA).
   http://www.emra.org/

2. Council of Emergency Medicine Residency Directors (CORD) Testing Web site. Got to pay for it.
   http://www.emtests.com/Default.htm

3. The Electronic Residency Application Service (ERAS)
   http://www.aamc.org/audienceeras.htm

4. Fellowship and Residency Electronic Interactive Database Online (FREIDA).
   http://www.ama-assn.org/ama/pub/category/2997.html

5. The SAEM Residency Vacancy Service.
   http://www.saem.org/saemdnn/Home/Communities/Residents/ResidencyVacancyService/tabid/152/Default.aspx

6. SAEM Resident Home Page. Great resource for residents.
   http://www.saem.org/saemdnn/Home/Communities/Residents/tabid/60/Default.aspx

7. Emergency Medicine Page. Keith's emergency medicine page—a must-read site!
   http://www.pitt.edu/~kconover/emed.htm

8. The Accreditation Council for Graduate Medical Education (ACGME). Say hi to mama.
   http://www.acgme.org/acWebsite/home/home.asp

9. **National Association of Residents and Interns.**
   http://www.nari-assn.com/index.html

10. **Meditrek.com.** Medical residency program management system.
    http://www.meditrek.com/default.htm

11. **FindAResident.** Powerful Web-based search tool to help you find open
    residency and fellowship positions.
    http://www.aamc.org/students/findaresident/start.htm

12. **Do Not Forget to Ask.** Advices on what to ask during residency interview.
    http://www.aamc.org/members/osr/residencyquestions.pdf

13. **Frequently Asked Questions about EM Residency.** Good overview.
    http://www.med.umich.edu/em/education/medstudents/FAQ's.htm

14. **eResidency.** Focused on the effective and efficient management of
    academic residency training programs.
    http://www.eresidency.net/

27. Toxicology

1. **The Agency for Toxic Substances and Disease Registry (ATSDR).**
    Great online resource.
    http://www.atsdr.cdc.gov/

2. **American College of Medical Toxicology. Great site.**
    http://www.acmt.net/main/contact.asp

3. **American Association of Poison Control Centers**. Electronic continuing
    education for specialists in poison information.
    http://www.urmc.rochester.edu/urmc/AAPCC/Welcome.htm

4. **Medical Management Guidelines for Acute Chemical Exposures**.
    CDC Wonder.
    **http://aepo-xdv-www.epo.cdc.gov/wonder/prevguid/p0000016/
    p0000016.asp**

5. **Managing Hazardous Materials Incidents Volume II, Hospital
    Emergency Departments (U.S. Department of Human Services).**
    **http://aepo-xdv-www.epo.cdc.gov/wonder/prevguid/p0000019/
    p0000019.asp**

6. **The Rocky Mountain Poison & Drug Center.** A medical information
    center.
    http://www.rmpdc.org/callcenter/index.cfm

7. **Toxicology Literature Online (TOXLINE)**. References from toxicology
    literature.
    http://toxnet.nlm.nih.gov/cgi-bin/sis/htmlgen?TOXLINE

8. **The Extension Toxicology Network (EXTOXNET).** Provides a variety of information about pesticides.
    http://extoxnet.orst.edu/

9. **Management of Chemical Warfare Agents Causalities.** A book to buy.
    http://members.aol.com/hbpub2/index.htm

10. **The Toxikon Multimedia Project.** The best site ever—a must-have!
    http://www.uic.edu/com/er/toxikon/index.htm

11. **Index of Poisonous Plants.**
    http://www.botanical.com/botanical/mgmh/poison.html

12. **Clinical Toxinology Resources Web site.** A premier site for information on venomous animals and poisonous animals.
    http://www.toxinology.com/fusebox.cfm?staticaction=generic_static_files/about_site.html

13. **Welcome to ToxTown.** An introduction to toxic chemicals and environmental health risks.
    http://toxtown.nlm.nih.gov/

14. **Poisoning and Toxicology Databases.** An amazing source of information!
    http://www.mednets.com/index.cfm/fuseaction/ articles_emergency_medicine_databases_search_engines_semerg

28. Ultrasound in ED

1. **American Emergency Ultrasonographic Society.**
    http://www.healthboard.com/websites/Detailed/48717.html

2. **EMCRIT**. Great introduction to U.S.—a must-read!
    http://www.emcrit.org/ultrasound/ultraindex.htm

3. **Emergency Medicine Ultrasound**. Discussion board.
    http://emultrasound.com

4. **Emergency Ultrasound.** ACEP Bookstore.
    http://www2.acep.org/bookstore/index.cfm?go=product.detail&id=10042

5. **Section of Emergency Ultrasound (ACEP).**
    http://www.acep.org/webportal/membercenter/sections/ultra/

6. **International Emergency Medicine Ultrasound**. Good site with great
    technical support.
    http://Vwww.usc.edu/schools/medicine/departments/emergency_medicine/international/Pages/ultrasound.html

7. **Introduction to Emergency Ultrasound**. A review of justifications,
    indications, and significant findings.
    http://www.dcmsonline.org/jax-edicine/1999journals/march99/ultrasound.htm

8. **Emergency Ultrasound**. Good images.
    http://www.smbs.buffalo.edu/emed/emed/ultrasound.html

9. **Ultrasound Database form Level 1 Trauma Center**. Awesome images collection.
http://www.hcmcem.com/us

10. **Implementing an Emergency Medicine Ultrasound Program (SAEM).**
http://www.saem.org/download/stahmer.pdf#search='emergency%20medicine%20ultrasound

11. **The ultimate ECHO-guide**. CD-ROM.
http://www.medicalamazon.com/15436.html

12. **Ultrasonography, Abdominal**. Read the article.
http://www.emedicine.com/emerg/topic621.htm

13. **Interesting Ultrasound Cases**. From UCSF.
http://ultrasound.ucsf.edu/USCases.html

14. **ARMDS (The Ultrasound Choice).**
http://www.ardms.org/index.htm

15. **Journal of Clinical Ultrasound.**
http://www3.interscience.wiley.com/cgi-bin/jhome/32273

16. **Interesting Ultrasound Cases**. From UCSF.
http://ultrasound.ucsf.edu/USCases.html

29. Specialties

I. Dermatology

1. **Dermatology Image Database.**
   http://tray.dermatology.uiowa.edu/DermImag.htm

2. **Dermatology Atlas.**
   http://www.meddean.luc.edu/lumen/MedEd/medicine/dermatology
   /title.htm

3. **The Electronic Textbook of Dermatology.**
   http://telemedicine.org/stamford.htm

4. **Dermatology Differential Diagnosis by Morphology**. Great resource.
   http://tray.dermatology.uiowa.edu/DDX-Morph.html#DDX

5. **Dermatology Image Atlas.** Images and links.
   http://www.dermatlas.org/derm

II. Ophthalmology

1. **Handbook of Ocular Disease Management.**
   http://www.revoptom.com/handbook/hbhome.htm

2. **Eyeorbit.gov**. The official eye site for everyone.
   http://www.eyeorbit.org/

III. Orthopedics

1. **Musculoskeletal Radiology of Fractures.**
    http://www.gentili.net/fracturemain.asp

2. **Wheeless' Textbook of Orthopaedics**. The best resource ever.
    http://www.wheelessonline.com

3. **Clinical Case Presentations**. From DuPont Hospital—orthopedics.
    http://gait.aidi.udel.edu/res695/homepage/pd_ortho/educate/
    clincase/clcasehp.htm

4. **Chirobase: Your Skeptical Guide to Chiropractics.**
    http://www.chirobase.org

5. **Sports Medicine and Orthopedic Surgery.** Timely information for
    patients and providers.
    http://www.emedx.com/

6. WorldOrtho—the World of Orthopaedics, Trauma, and Sports Medicine.
    http://www.worldortho.com/

IV. Palliative Care

1. **End of Life/Palliative Education Resource Center.** Foster the continued
    development of palliative care education.
    http://www.eperc.mcw.edu/

2. **The End of Life Care Research Program.**
    http://depts.washington.edu/eolcare

3. **Welcome to the EPEC Project. Education in palliative and end-of-
    life care.**
    http://epec.net/EPEC/webpages/index.cfm

V. Surgery and Trauma

1. **Trauma.org**. One of the best sites—a must-read.
    http://www.trauma.org/

2. **Trauma Surgery Site**. Educational site with lots of procedures.
   http://www.simulab.com/TraumaSurgery.htm

3. **Trauma Practice Guidelines.** A must-have.
   http://www.east.org/tpg.html

4. **Trauma X-Ray Collection.** Nice selection of the x-rays.
   http://www.swsahs.nsw.gov.au/livtrauma/education/xray.asp

VI. Wilderness Medicine

1. **Welcome to SOLO Wilderness Medicine**. Dedicated to teaching wilderness and emergency medicine.
   http://www.soloschools.com/about.html

2. **Wilderness Emergency Medical Services Institute-provides medical care to patients in the specialized prehospital situations.**
   http://www.wemsi.org/

3. **Wilderness Medical Associates.** Leading the world in teaching wilderness and rescue medicine.
   http://www.wildmed.com/

4. **National Conferences on Wilderness Medicine (March 2006)**
   http://www.wilderness-medicine.com/

5. **The High Altitude Medicine Guide.** Very good resource.
   http://www.high-altitude-medicine.com/

Medical Organizations and Useful Links

A

1. **AirMed International.** Ambulance and air medical.
   http://www.airmed.com/amMain/main.asp

2. **Air Medical Physician Association.**
   http://www.ampa.org/

3. **Ambulansforum.**
   http://www.ambulansforum.se/

4. **American Ambulance Association.**
   http://www.the-aaa.org/

5. **Association of Air Medical Services.**
   http://www.aams.org//AM/Template.cfm?Section=Home

6. **Commission on Accreditation of Medical Transport.**
   http://www.camts.org/

7. **Commission on Accredited Ambulance Services.**
   http://www.caas.org/

8. **Flightweb**. Air medical site.
   http://www.flightweb.com/index.php

9. **National Academy of Emergency Dispatch.**
   http://www.emergencydispatch.org/

10. **Royal Flying Doctor Service of Australia.**
    http://www.saem.org/
    http://www.flyingdoctor.net/

11. **Academic Medicine**. Journal of AAMC.
    http://www.academicmedicine.org/

12. **Access Medicine Services**. Immediate access to medical information resources.
    http://genetics.accessmedicine.com/amed/public/amed_order/order.html

13. **Accreditation Council for Graduate Medical Education (ACGME).**
    http://www.acgme.org/acWebsite/home/home.asp

14. **Agency of Health Care Research and Quality**. Advancing excellence in health care.
    http://www.ahrq.gov/

15. **AIDSMEDS Online**. HIV+ owned and operated site—great resource of information.
    http://www.aidsmeds.com/

16. **ALERTS**. Automated live e-health—a must-see!
    http://www.pharmacon.com/products.html

17. **AHIMA**. The premier association of health information management (HIM) professionals.
    http://www.ahima.org/about/about.asp

18. **American Heart Association**. Speaks for itself.
    http://www.americanheart.org/

19. **American Hospital Association**. Represents and serves all types of hospitals, health care networks, and their patients and communities.
    http://www.hospitalconnect.com/hospitalconnect_app/index.jsp

20. **American Medical Informatics Association**. An organization of leaders shaping the future of health information technology.
    http://www.amia.org/mbrcenter

21. **American Nurses Association**. Official site for the nurses.
    http://www.nursingworld.org/

22. **Alphabetic List of Specific Diseases/Disorders.**
    http://www.mic.ki.se/Diseases/Alphalist.html

23. **Ambulatory Pediatric Association**. Fosters the health of children, adolescents, and families.
    http://www.ambpeds.org/

24. **American Association for Health Education**. Serves professionals in the following settings: health care, community, agency, business, school (K-12), and higher education.
    http://www.med.usf.edu/~kmbrown/AAHE.htm

25. **The American Association for the Surgery of Trauma.** Promotes scientific information regarding all phases of the care of the trauma patient.
    http://www.aast.org/

26. **American Board of Medical Specialties.**
    http://www.abms.org/

27. **American Society of Law, Medicine & Ethics.** Best educational information at the intersection of law, medicine, and ethics.
    http://www.aslme.org/about/index.php

28. **American Pain Society**. The issues related to pain including clinical and basic research, patient care, education, and health policy.
    http://www.ampainsoc.org/

29. **Association of American Medical Colleges**. You must know this site.
    http://www.aamc.org/

30. **The Asthma Information Outreach Project**. Created to meet the information needs of asthma providers and researchers in New York City by providing them with library and Web services.
    http://www.asthma-nyc.org/

31. **American College of Physicians**. Everything about internal medicine.
    http://www.acponline.org/

B

1. **Bandolier**. Evidence-based thinking.
   http://www.jr2.ox.ac.uk/bandolier

2. **The Body Pro.com.** The online resource dedicated to the needs of HIV/AIDS health care professionals.
   http://www.thebodypro.com/index.shtml

3. **Bulletin of World Health Organization.**
   http://www.who.int/bulletin/en

C

1. **Cancer Online Resources**. Great site.
   http://www.acor.org/

2. **Centers for Disease Control and Prevention (CDC).** Got to know this site.
   http://www.cdc.gov/page.do

3. **ClinicalTrials.gov**. Provides regularly updated information about federally and privately supported clinical research in human volunteers.
   http://www.clinicaltrials.gov/

4. **CNN-Health**. Useful updates and health news.
   http://www.cnn.com/HEALTH

5. **The Cochrane Collaboration.** The reliable source of evidence in health care.
   http://www.cochrane.org/

6. **Center Watch Clinical Trials Listing Service**. Information about clinical research.
   http://www.centerwatch.com/

7. **National electronic Library for Health**. Provides a regularly updated guide to evidence about the effectiveness of care.
   http://www.nelh.nhs.uk/clinical_evidence.asp

8. **Contraception.net—Contraception Resource Center**. Great site.
   http://www.contraception.net/

9. **The Council of Emergency Medicine Residency Directors (CORD).**
    A scientific and educational organization.
    http://www.cordem.org/

10. **Council of Medical Specialty Societies (CMSS).** A unique forum in
    U.S. medicine.
    http://www.cmss.org/index.cfm

D

I. Disaster Medicine

1. **American Red Cross.**
    http://www.redcross.org/

2. **Comprehensive Emergency Service Search & Research Tool.**
    http://www.psasb.us/

3. **Disaster Homepage.**
    http://mediccom.org/public/default.htm

4. **Doctors Without Borders.**
    http://www.dwb.org/

5. **Emergency Preparedness Information exchange.**
    http://epix.hazard.net/

6. **FEMA.**
    http://www.fema.gov/

7. **International Medical Corps.**
    http://www.imcworldwide.org/index.shtml

8. **National Association for Search and Rescue.**
    http://www.nasar.org/nasar/

9. **National Institute for Urban Search and Rescue.**
    http://niusr.org/go/site/969/

10. **National Safety Council.**
    http://www.nsc.org/

11. **Office of Emergency Preparedness.**
    http://www.oep-ndms.dhhs.gov/

12. **RapidReach.** Emergency Notification.
    http://www.enera.com/

13. **Rock Medical Web Site.**
    http://www.rockmed.org/

14. **SAR Information.**
    http://www.sarinfo.bc.ca/

15. **World Association for Disaster and Emergency Medicine.**
    http://wadem.medicine.wisc.edu/

16. **Disaster Medical Assistance Team.**
    http://mediccom.org/public/default.htm

17. **Drug Enforcement Administration (DEA).**
    http://www.usdoj.gov/dea/index.htm

18. **Department of Health and Human Services.**
    http://www.os.dhhs.gov/

19. **DOCLINE.** The National Library of Medicine's automated interlibrary loan (ILL) request routing and referral system.
    http://www.nlm.nih.gov/pubs/factsheets/docline.html

20. **The Doctors' Page.** The Web site specifically designed for the practicing physician.
    http://doctorspage.net/

E

1. **Emerging Infectious Diseases.** Published monthly by the National Center for Infectious Diseases, Centers for Disease Control and Prevention (CDC).
    http://www.cdc.gov/ncidod/eid/index.htm

2.   **ECARE® Online**. A powerful resource designed to help you with a wide variety of everyday tasks.
     http://www.ecare.com/

3.   **e-Discharge.** A process management solution that streamlines the discharge process.
     http://www.edischarge.com/login.cfm

4.   **Educational Commission for Foreign Medical Graduate (ECFMG).**
     http://www.ecfmg.org/

5.   **eHANYS**. The electronic channel for marketplace solutions designed by the Healthcare Association of New York State (HANYS).
     http://www.ehanys.com/

6.   **Education in Legal Medicine (ELM).** Provides a unified curriculum for health care providers.
     http://www.elmexchange.com/

7.   **Electronic Network Systems Inc. (ENS)**. Pioneered the rapid evolution of electronic data interchange (EDI) and medical reimbursements within the health care industry.
     http://www.edss.com/

8.   **Elsevier Science Direct**. The ultimate scientific, technical, and medical resource.
     http://www.elsevier.com/wps/find/homepage.cws_home

9.   **eMedNY**. The name of the new electronic Medicaid system of New York State.
     http://www.emedny.org/

10. **eResidency Home Page.** Focused on the effective and efficient management of academic residency training programs.
     http://www.eresidency.net/

11. **Electronic Medical Outcomes**. Automates nearly every aspect of outcomes data collection.
     http://www.emedoutcomes.org/

12. **The Eastern Association for the Surgery of Trauma.**
     http://www.east.org/

F

1. **Federal Government Health Portal.** A portal to the Web sites of the
    U.S. Department of Health and Human Services (HHS).
    http://www.health.gov/

2. **Federation of State Medical Boards.**
    http://www.fsmb.org/

3. **FIRSTConsult.com.** Unique content, specially written for rapid access
    and fast retrieval at the point of care.
    http://www.firstconsult.com/home/framework/ fs_main.htm?ip_
    auth=true&

4. **The Food Allergy & Anaphylaxis Network (FAAN).** Serves as the
    communication link between the patient and others.
    http://www.foodallergy.org/about.html

5. **FREIDA Online**. Information about residency and fellowship programs.
    http://www.ama-assn.org/ama/pub/category/2997.html

6. **Fire Department and EMS Educational Sites**. Have a blast!
    http://www.mindspring.com/~katy/CarrWilson/search.html

G

1. **GME Toolkit.** Premier data management solution that assists residency
    programs.
    http://www.gmetoolkit.com/

2. **Greater New York Hospital Association (GNYHA).** Trade association
    representing more than 250 nonprofit hospitals and continuing care
    facilities
    http://www.gnyha.org/

H

II. HAZMAT

1. Advanced Hazmat Life Support.
   http://www.ahls.org/ahls/ecs/main/ahls_home.html

2. American Association of Poison Control Centers.
   http://www.aapcc.org/

3. California Department of Pesticide Regulation.
   http://www.cdpr.ca.gov/

4. Canadian Center for Occupational Health & Safety.
   http://www.ccohs.ca/oshanswers/

5. ChemFinder WebServe.
   http://chemfinder.cambridgesoft.com/

6. Clinical Pharmacology Online.
   http://www.clinicalpharmacology.com/Default.asp

7. Divers Alert Network.
   http://www.diversalertnetwork.org/

8. **EXTOXNET.** The Extension Toxicology Network.
   http://extoxnet.orst.edu/

9. Hazmat DB.
   http://www.atsdr.cdc.gov/hazdat.html#A3.1.2a

10. MSDS Sheets from Oxford University.
    http://joule.pcl.ox.ac.uk/MSDS/

11. National Hazards Center (University of Colorado).
    http://www.colorado.edu/hazards/

12. OSHA Bloodborne Pathogens.
    http://www.osha.gov/SLTC/bloodbornepathogens/index.html

13. **Snakebite Protocols.**
     http://drdavidson.ucsd.edu/Portals/0/index.htm

14. **Tetanus Page.**
     http://www.cyberhorse.net.au/csl/tetanus.htm

15. **Wilderness Medical Society.**
     http://www.wms.org/

H

1. **Handheldmed.com.** Browse, try, and buy at the e-book store.
    http://www.handheldmed.com/Site.New/Pages.php?p=welcome

2. **HealthStream.** Health care learning network.
    http://www.healthstream.com/index.htm

3. **Hardin MD-great medical links.** A must-see.
    http://www.lib.uiowa.edu/hardin/md

4. **Health Information Library.** Great links.
    http://www.nlm.nih.gov/hinfo.html

5. **The Healthcare Association of New York State (HANYS).** Provides
    hospital members with access to quality supplies at excellent prices.
    http://www.hanys.org/communications/pr/pr102604a.cfm

6. **HealthFirst.** The leader in providing emergency kits.
    http://www.healthfirst.com/Default.aspx

7. **HealthSTAR.** Health games and info for teens.
    http://www.healthstar.com.au/

8. **HIPAA.** Everything you need to know.
    http://www.hipaa.org/

9. **HIVinSITE.** Comprehensive information about HIV/AIDS.
    http://hivinsite.ucsf.edu/

I

1. **Institute for Safe Medication Practices (ISMP).** Reducing patient harm from preventable adverse drug events.
    http://www.ismp.org/

2. **InteliHealth.** Comprehensive collection of health consumer information.
    http://www.intelihealth.com/IH/ihtIH/WSIHW000/408/408.
    html?k=menux408x408

J

1. **Jacobi Hyperbaric.** Indications and applications for hyperbaric oxygen therapy.
    http://www.jacobi-hyperbaric.com/

2. **JCAHO.** Supposed to be our friend.
    http://www.jcaho.org/

3. **The Junior Fellows Program.** Designed to stimulate middle and high school students' interest in health, science, medicine, and research.
    http://www.juniorfellows.org/

K

1. **Kaplan Medical.** Test for medical professionals.
    http://www.kaptest.com/med_home.jhtml

L

1. **Lab Tests online.** A public resource on clinical lab testing.
    http://www.labtestsonline.org/

2. **The LANCET.** International journal of medical science and practice.
    http://www.thelancet.com/

3. **Lippincott Williams & Wilkins.** Offering specialized publications and software for physicians, nurses, students, and specialized clinicians.
    http://www.lww.com/

4. **LinkedIn.com**. Enables connections and offers jobs listings.
   http://www.linkedin.com/

M

1. **Magnacare.** A site dedicated to medical products.
   http://www.magnacare.com.au

2. **Mayo Clinic.** Tool for healthier lives.
   http://www.mayoclinic.com

3. **MDLinx**. A network of several dozen professional Web sites for physicians.
   http://www.woodbournesolutions.com/clients/MDLinx.cfm

4. **The MEDEM network**. Premier physician-patient communications network.
   http://www.medem.com/

5. **MEDERRORS.com**. Devoted to providing information on medication errors and adverse drug events in hospitals.
   http://www.mederrors.com/

6. **MedTerms Medical Dictionary**. An online medical dictionary.
   http://www.medterms.com/script/main/hp.asp

7. **MerckMedicus.** More relevant search results from specific resources with time-saving efficiency.
   http://www.merckmedicus.com/pp/us/hcp/hcp_home.jsp

8. **Medicare Interactive (MI)**. One-stop source for information about health care rights, options, and benefits.
   http://www.medicareinteractive.org/

9. **Medical News & Weblog Aggregator**. Medical news feeds and blogging—a great site.
   http://www.medlogs.com/

10. **Medical Links out of NYC**. Nice list.
    http://www.nyc.gov/html/hhc/qhn/html/links.html

11. **Medical Mnemonics**. For those who cannot remember things.
http://www.medicalmnemonics.com/

N

III. **North American Organizations for Emergency Medicine, Trauma, and Critical Care**

1. **American Academy of Experts in Traumatic Stress.**
http://www.aaets.org/

2. **American Academy of Urgent Care Medicine.**
http://www.urgentcaremedicine.org/

3. **American Association of Critical Care Nurses.**
http://www.aacn.org/

4. **American Association for the Surgery of Trauma.**
http://www.aast.org/

5. **American Board of Emergency Medicine.**
http://www.abem.org/public/

6. **American College of Osteopathic Emergency Physicians.**
http://www.acoep.org/

7. **American College of Preventive Medicine.**
http://www.acpm.org/

8. **American College of Surgeons.**
http://www.facs.org/

9. **American Forensic Nurses.**
http://www.amrn.com/

10. **American Health Informatics Management Association.**
http://www.ahima.org/

11. **American Osteopathic Board of Emergency Medicine.**
http://www.aobem.org/

12. **American Society of Emergency Radiology.**
    http://www.erad.org/

13. **Association of Emergency Physicians.**
    http://www.aep.org/

14. **California EMS.**
    http://www.emsa.cahwnet.gov/

15. **Canadian Association of Critical Care Nurses.**
    http://www.caccn.ca/new/

16. **Canadian Association of Emergency Physicians.**
    http://www.caep.ca/

17. **Center for Rural Emergency Medicine (WVU).**
    http://www.hsc.wvu.edu/crem/

18. **Council of Emergency Medicine Resident Directors.**
    http://www.cordem.org/

19. **Doctors Who Care**. A list of dedicated Web sites.
    http://www.doctorswhocare.org/

20. **Eastern Association for Surgery of Trauma.**
    http://www.east.org/

21. **Emergency Medicine Network**. Involves 180 medical centers.
    http://www.emnet-usa.org/

22. **Emergency Medicine Residents Association.**
    http://www.emra.org/

23. **Emergency Nurses Association.**
    http://www.ena.org/

24. **EMS Administrators Association of California.**
    http://www.emsaac.com/

25. **Florida Association of EMS Educators.**
http://www.faemse.org/

26. **Foundation for Education and Research in Neurological Emergencies.**
http://www.ferne.org/
http://www.injurypreventionweb.org/

27. **Institute of Critical Care Medicine.**
http://www.911research.org/

28. **JCAHO.**
http://www.jointcommission.org/

29. **Journal Club on the Web**. Old but still deserves to be looked at.
http://www.journalclub.org/

30. **Medical Group Management Association.**
http://www.mgma.com/

31. **National Association for Ambulatory Care.**
http://www.urgentcare.org/

32. **National Association of Emergency Medicine Educators.**
http://www.naemse.org/

33. **National Association EMS Physicians.**
http://www.naemsp.org/

34. **National Association of Emergency Medicine Technicians.**
http://www.naemt.org/

35. **National Association of State EMS Directors.**
http://www.naemsp.org/

36. **National Center for Early Defibrillation.**
http://www.early-defib.org/

37. **National Center for Emergency Medicine Informatics.**
http://ncemi.org/

38. National Collegiate EMS Foundation
    http://www.ncemsf.org/

39. National Council of State EMS Training Coordinators.
    http://www.ncsemstc.org/

40. National Emergency Medicine Association.
    http://www.nemahealth.org/

41. National Highway Traffic Safety Administration.
    http://www.nhtsa.dot.gov/

42. National Rural Health Association.
    http://www.nrharural.org/

43. National Society of EMS Educators.
    http://www.naemse.org/

44. National Stroke Association.
    http://www.stroke.org/site/PageServer?pagename=HOME

45. New York State EMS Office.
    http://www.health.state.ny.us/nysdoh/ems/main.htm

46. Orthopaedic Trauma Association.
    http://www.ota.org/

47. Physicians for a Violence-Free Society.
    http://www.aast.org/pvs.html

48. Royal Society of Medicine.
    http://www.roysocmed.ac.uk/

49. Society of Critical Care Medicine.
    http://www.sccm.org/sccm

50. Society of Emergency Medicine PAs.
    http://www.sempa.org/

51. **Society of Trauma Nurses.**
    http://www.traumanursesoc.org/

52. **Texas Department of Health EMS.**
    http://www.tdh.state.tx.us/hcqs/ems/emshome.htm

53. **Urgent Care Association of America.**
    http://www.ucaoa.org/

54. **Virginia EMS.**
    http://www.vdh.state.va.us/oems/index.asp

55. **New Innovations**. Residency management site.
    http://www.new-innov.com/

56. **New York Online to Health (NOAH).**
    http://www.noah-health.org/

57. **National Institute on Drug Abuse (NIDA).**
    http://www.nida.nih.gov/

58. **National Library of Medicine.**
    http://www.nlm.nih.gov/

O

27. **OSHA**. To ensure the safety and health of America's workers.
    http://www.osha.gov/

P

1. **Patient Education Institute**. An established provider of patient and
    health education systems and software.
    http://www.patient-education.com/

2. **Pharmacological Reviews**. Great updates
    http://pharmrev.aspetjournals.org/

3. **Point of Care Testing Information Online**. Most comprehensive resource site.
   http://www.pointofcare.net/

4. **Postgraduate Medicine.** Great journal to read.
   http://www.postgradmed.com/

5. **Prison Health Services**. Founder of the privately managed correctional health care field.
   http://www.prisonhealth.com/

Q

IV. Quality and Patient Safety Links

1. **ACEP Quality Improvement & Patient Safety.**
   http://www.acep.org/webportal/membercenter/sections/qips/

2. **Quality To Improve Patient Safety (QTIPS).**
   http://www.acep.org/qtips/

3. **Agency for Health Care Research and Quality.**
   http://www.ahrq.gov/

4. **Physician Consortium for Performance Improvement.**
   http://www.ama-assn.org/ama/pub/category/2946.html

5. **Joint Commission on Accreditation of Healthcare Organizations (JACHO).**
   http://www.jointcommission.org/

6. **The National Committee for Quality Assurance(NCQA).**
   http://www.ncqa.org/

7. **The Emergency Medicine Patient Safety Foundation. Dedicated to improving patient safety in emergency medicine.**
   http://www.empsf.org/index.asp

8. MedWatch. Your Internet gateway for timely safety information on drugs and other medical products.
    http://www.fda.gov/medwatch/

9. The Institute of Medicine. It serves as adviser to the nation to improve health.
    http://www.iom.edu/

10. The Institute for Health Care Improvement.
    http://www.ihi.org/ihi

11. The Institute for Safe Medication Practices.
    http://www.ismp.org/

12. The National Patient Safety Foundation.
    http://www.npsf.org/

13. The Society of Chest Pain Centers.
    http://www.scpcp.org/

R

1. ED Physician. With 1,200 emergency medicine and urgent care jobs in all states.
    http://www.edphysician.com/

2. EmCare. Nation's leading provider of emergency care.
    http://www.emcare.com/

3. Emergency Physician Jobs. Really finds the job.
    http://www.emergencyphysicianjobs.com/

4. Emergency Physicians Monthly. Online resource and blog for physicians.
    http://www.epmonthly.com/

5. ERWork. Over 1,800 clients (hospitals, clinics, and private practices)
    http://www.nhrphysician.com/

6. **Emergency Practice Association**. Practice management service.
    http://www.epamidwest.com/

S

1. **Scientific American Medicine Online**. Most up-to-date clinical information.
    http://www.ramex.com/title.asp?id=1618

2. **The Society of Forensic Toxicologists.**
    http://www.soft-tox.org/

3. **3M Littmann Stethoscopes.** A trusted leader in auscultation technology.
    http://www.3m.com/us/healthcare/professionals/littmann/jhtml

4. **Shoes and Clogs for Health Professionals.**
    http://www.medshoes.com/

5. **Stumps, Marking Devices, and Indoor Signs (Logan Stamp Works).**
    http://www.loganstamp.com/

6. **Stat Medical Supply Company. Good luck shopping.**
    http://www.statmedical.com/

T

1. **The Body PRO (HIV/AIDS Resource for Health Professionals).**
    http://www.thebodypro.com/index.shtml

V

V. **RECRUITERS**

1. **VaccineShoppe**. Good information and ordering site.
    http://www.vaccineshoppe.com/

Sergey's Special—IMG Resources

International Medical Graduates

1. **IMGPREP.** Provides assistance and counseling for IMGs in USA.
    http://www.imgprep.com/scramble/

2. **International Medical Graduates Match and Scramble Services.**
    http://www.imgresidency.com/

3. **International Medical Graduate Institute.**
    http://www.imgi.net/

4. **Canadian International Medical Graduate Web site.**
    http://members.tripod.com/donalda13

5. **The International Medical Graduate Page Index.**
    http://members.aol.com/AkramKhan/IMG/Page1.html

6. **American Dream Abroad.**
    http://www.americandreamabroad.com/ourMission.html

7. **The International Medical Association (IMA).**
    http://members.tripod.com/~IMGA/index.html

8. **International Medical Graduates.** Clinical rotations and residency in USA.
    http://gmcgroup.org/index.asp

9. **International Medical Graduate Web Sites.** Very useful links.
    http://www.visalaw.com/IMG/ethnic.html

10. **IMG Society's Online**. Built to bring together all of the diverse international medical graduate.
    http://www.imgsociety.org/

11. **IMG Guides**. For international students.
    http://emran3.tripod.com/imglinks.htm

12. **ECFMG**. Information booklets.
    http://www.pages.drexel.edu/~dmd42/2003ib/ibgrad.html

13. **Clinical Medicine Program.** Rotations for graduates
    http://www.gmcgroup.org/cmp.asp

14. **Edvisors.com (International: Foreign Medical Schools)**. Multiple useful links.
    http://www.edvisors.com/International/Foreign_Medical_Schools/index.html

15. **International Medical Placement Ltd.**
    http://www.intlmedicalplacement.com/internationalPhysician.html

16. **Kaplan Medical**. Best tutorials and courses for IMGs.
    http://www.kaptest.com/usmle

17. **International Medical Graduates in the USA (Graham McMahon)**. Absolutely the best!
    http://www.internationaldoc.com/

18. **Match A Resident**. Customized residency reports.
    http://www.matcharesident.com/main.php

19. **Welcome to Electronic Residency**. Allows the fastest submission of your electronic application during the Match, Scramble, and Post-Scramble seasons in one click.
    http://www.electronicresidency.com

20. **Medgraduate.com.** For FMG—a meeting place for foreign medical graduates.
    http://www.medgraduate.com/?gclid=CPGJ_M7uzIgCFQVvHgod cwb7KQ

21. **List of Friendly Hospitals for Residency.** For IMG.
     http://www.medgraduate.com/resfriendly.php

22. **InfoIMG.** Dedicated to providing information to international medical
     graduates (IMGs).
     http://www.infoimg.com/

23. **USMLE FORUM.** Great site!
     http://usmleforum.org/

24. **FMG America (Foreign Medical Graduates U.S. Residency Counseling).**
     http://www.fmgamerica.com/